Central Venous Pressure

Central Venous Pressure

Its Clinical Use and Role in Cardiovascular Dynamics

W. J. Russell
M.B., B.S., F.F.A.R.C.S.
Wellcome Research Fellow, Department of Anaesthetics, Royal Postgraduate Medical School, Hammersmith Hospital, London

Butterworths

ENGLAND:	BUTTERWORTH & CO. (PUBLISHERS) LTD. LONDON: 88 Kingsway, WC2B 6AB
AUSTRALIA:	BUTTERWORTHS PTY. LTD. SYDNEY: 586 Pacific Highway, 2067 MELBOURNE: 343 Little Collins Street, 3000 BRISBANE: 240 Queen Street, 4000
CANADA:	BUTTERWORTH & CO. (CANADA) LTD. TORONTO: 14 Curity Avenue, 374
NEW ZEALAND:	BUTTERWORTHS OF NEW ZEALAND LTD. WELLINGTON: 26–28 Waring Taylor Street, 1
SOUTH AFRICA:	BUTTERWORTH & CO. (SOUTH AFRICA) (PTY.) LTD. DURBAN: 152–154 Gale Street

Suggested U.D.C. Number: 612.144

Suggested Additional Numbers: 616.12–008.341

ISBN 0 407 13270 8

Text set in 11 pt. Photon Times, printed by photolithography, and bound in Great Britain at The Pitman Press, Bath

Contents

Preface

This monograph is not a report of original experimental work but an explanation of central venous pressure for clinicians. It has four objectives: to explain the part played by the central venous pressure in cardiovascular dynamics; to discuss the clinical need to measure central venous pressure; to describe the apparatus and its use; and to discuss the interpretation of the measurements. This, I hope, will provide a guide to the management of patients with cardiovascular instability.

I wish to thank Professor J. G. Robson, Professor M. K. Sykes and my colleagues at the Royal Postgraduate Medical School and Hammersmith Hospital for their encouragement and suggestions during the writing of this monograph. I am also very grateful to my wife for much of the typing and preparation of the manuscript.

The kind permission of Professor A. C. Guyton, the American Journal of Physiology, Professor M. K. Sykes, the Annals of the Royal College of Surgeons of England, Professor G. S. Moss, the Annals of Surgery, Dr. T. Boulton and St. Bartholomew's Hospital Journal is acknowledged for the use of their illustrations.

W.J.R.

I
Central Venous Pressure in Cardiovascular Dynamics

The Cardiovascular System

Introduction

The first man to measure central venous pressure was Stephen Hales, in the 1st decade of the 18th century, although the exact date of his first experiment is uncertain. This measurement may have been made, while they were both at Cambridge, in co-operation with his friend William Stuckley, who was studying medicine there. In this first experiment they probably used a dog. Hales' better known observations on the venous pressure of mares were made later when he was vicar at Teddington (Clark-Kennedy, 1929). His years at Cambridge had given him a clear understanding of hydrostatics and so he was careful to refer his pressure observations to the level of the left ventricle. This set an excellent example for those who were to follow but unfortunately, even today, venous pressures are sometimes quoted without the reference level being stated. Hales not only measured the pressure at the internal jugular vein during his experiments, but he also observed that the pressure rose when the mare struggled.

These observations remained isolated for about 170 years. Then, in the later part of the 19th century, it was noted that venous pressure altered with changes in blood volume (Cohnheim and Lichtheim, 1877) and that it influenced the work of the heart (Howell and Donaldson, 1884).

During the past 50 years our understanding of the physiology of the heart and of the venous return has steadily improved. With this better insight we have been more able to appreciate the significance of the central venous pressure and to see how it results from the interaction of the venous return and the cardiac function. However, central venous pressure is but one element in the juggling act of cardiovascular dynamics and its significance can be appreciated only when those dynamics are understood.

A convenient approach is to develop a model of the cardiovascular system. This model should not be too simple for it must adequately simulate the system, yet it must not be too complex or the behaviour of the model will not be understood and the vital insight into how the system works will be lost. When the dynamics are appreciated, variations in central venous pressure can be explained logically and the management of low output states can be approached rationally.

The cardiovascular system is a closed loop and a change in any part must have repercussions throughout the system. Normally, changes are perceived by specific receptors and counteracted through the autonomic nervous system. The chain of repercussions can be demonstrated by following the effect of infusing additional blood into the systemic veins. When blood is infused intravenously, the systemic volume is increased and the resistance of the venous side of systemic circulation diminishes. There is also a small rise in local venous pressure. Both these effects enhance the flow of blood back to the heart and this improved flow increases the pressure in the right atrium, the output of the right ventricle and pulmonary artery pressure. The increased pressure in the pulmonary artery increases flow through the pulmonary circulation which in turn increases the pulmonary venous pressure and the pressure in the left atrium. This atrial pressure change enhances the flow of blood into the left ventricle and thus increases the systemic arterial pressure. The systemic arterial pressure affects the capillary flow and the systemic venous flow. Thus, in time, a disturbance is felt all round the cardiovascular loop.

Although the vascular system is closed it is not rigid. It is sensitive to changes in pressure mainly because the ventricles, which pump the blood through the circulation, are sensitive to their filling pressure. Any pressure changes—particularly a change on the venous side of the heart—alter the performance of the ventricles. Thus the heart is a pressure-sensitive pump driving blood around the body.

For many purposes an adequate model of the system can be made if we assume that the right ventricular output effectively governs the left ventricular output and the pulmonary circulation can be ignored. This 'single pump' simplification means that only a two-part model is required; a heart and a systemic circulation. Much valuable insight into the function of the cardiovascular system can be gained from this simpler model.

The heart

Many studies have been made of mammalian cardiac function, both with isolated hearts and in intact animals. Each approach has its own special difficulties but a common result can be expressed briefly: increased atrial pressure produces increased ventricular output. This is sometimes called Starling's law of the heart (Starling, 1918). It has been studied mainly in animals but has been shown to occur also in man (Braunwald and Ross, 1964).

We can understand this effect if we assume each ventricle has two properties: (1) that it will pump onwards whatever volume fills it—that is, for a given rate and resistance the ventricular volume at the end of systole is always the same regardless of the volume at the end of diastole; (2) that in diastole the ventricle is a compliant chamber, the filling of which is governed by the pressure gradient from just within the atrioventricular valve to just outside the ventricular wall in the pericardial sac (Berglund, 1954). This filling pressure is illustrated in *Figure 1*. Normally, the pressure just outside the ventricle is the intrathoracic pressure. In normal circumstances, therefore, the filling pressure for the ventricle is closely approximated by the pressure difference between the atrium and the pleural space. The importance of the pressure just inside the atrioventricular valve is shown by the observation (Guyton and Greganti, 1956) that the pressure just inside the tricuspid valve was the best reference for ventricular filling and remained almost unchanged with changes in posture.

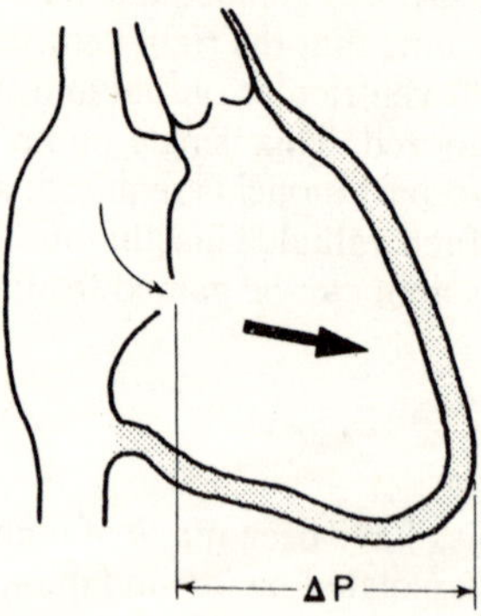

Figure 1. Diagram of the pressure gradient for ventricular filling. As the ventricle is a compliant chamber, it will fill until there is no pressure gradient between its interior and the atrium. The pressure across the ventricular wall is then balanced by the tension within the wall. In the dynamic situation some of the pressure between the atrioventricular valve and the pericardial space is taken up with the flow of blood into the distending ventricle. However, the statement that ventricular filling depends on the pressure gradient still remains true, although the relationship may not be a simple one

Any increase in pressure just outside the ventricle diminishes the pressure gradient. For example, fluid in the pericardium increases the pressure outside the ventricles and hinders ventricular filling (Spodick, 1967). If the pressure immediately outside the ventricle in the pericardial sac is constant, any increase in atrial pressure increases the pressure gradient and hence increases the ventricular filling. Thus increased atrial pressure increases the end-diastolic volume, the stroke volume and the cardiac output.

The ability of the ventricle to increase its output as the atrial pressure is increased can be demonstrated by a cardiac performance curve. The curve shows the response of the ventricle over a range of atrial pressures. The upper limit of the performance curve is only achieved by a high atrial pressure. A very low atrial pressure may produce almost no output. Thus the performance curve relates the ventricular filling pressure to the ventricular output, and in fact separate performance curves should apply to the right and left sides of the heart. Each curve (or pair) describes the heart under set conditions which are determined by the sympathetic and parasympathetic activity impinging on the heart and by the intrinsic quality of the ventricular muscle. The level of autonomic activity influences both heart rate and myocardial contractility and thus plays a major role in determining the ability of the heart to respond to the atrial pressure. Maximal sympathetic influence gives a high performance curve, while minimal sympathetic influence gives a low performance curve. A family of curves describe the possible performance of the heart under the widest range of conditions (*Figure 2*). Usually attention is focused on the highest performance curve as this is the one most deteriorated by disease. However, from the potential performance, the actual cardiac output is determined by the atrial pressure which fills the ventricle, and could be any amount between nothing and the upper limit of the performance curve.

The output of the heart depends upon the right atrial pressure and on the autonomic activity which is the main determinant of the cardiac performance curve. An increase in cardiac output could be achieved by an increase in right atrial pressure or an improvement in ventricular performance. Normally changes in cardiac output are achieved by adjustment of the autonomic nervous activity which changes the ventricular performance. These multiple levels of ventricular performance have been described as the Frank-Starling mechanism (Sarnoff, 1955; Fry, Braunwald and Cohen, 1960). This is probably the natural mechanism for regulating cardiac output in health, while the atrial pressure/ventricular output mechanism maintains the precise balance between the ventricles. In *Figure 2* this effective ventricular filling pressure is expressed as right atrial pressure, assuming a constant mean pressure in the pericardial sac.

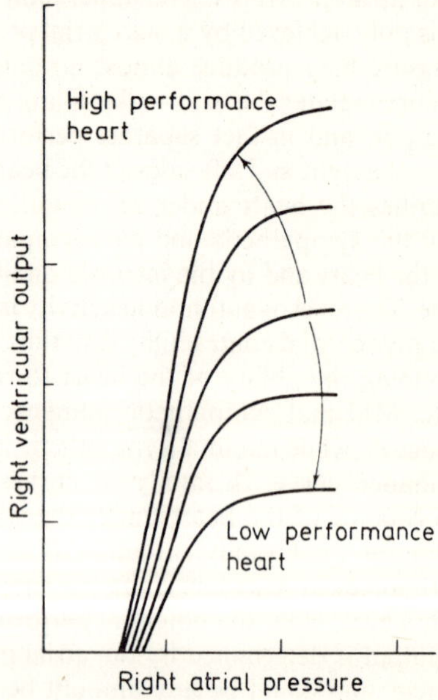

Figure 2. Diagram of Frank-Starling curves. The output increases as the right atrial pressure increases until a maximum is reached when further rises in right atrial pressure do not improve output (and may possibly diminish it). Increased sympathetic activity increases the sensitivity of the heart to right atrial pressure (high performance heart): there is a greater increase in output for the same right atrial pressure, and the maximum output is greater. Conversely, parasympathetic influences or myocardial damage reduce the sensitivity to atrial pressure and also cause a reduction in the maximum output

When the heart is beating slowly, the ventricle can fill to the atrial pressure well before atrial systole occurs; the volume in the right ventricle at the end of diastole is effectively governed by the right atrial pressure, and hence this pressure controls the stroke volume. As cardiac output is the product of the stroke volume and the heart rate, it would be determined by the heart rate alone if a given right atrial pressure produced a consistent stroke volume. A family of Frank–Starling curves would then be merely an expression of a succession of heart rates. A slow heart rate means the cardiac output would increase only modestly with an increase in atrial pressure and this could be expressed as a low performance curve (*Figure 2*). For example, at a rate of 60 beats/min a change in atrial pressure which produced a 10 ml increase in stroke volume would improve the cardiac output by 600 ml/min; at a rate of 120 beats/min, the same increase in stroke volume would improve the output by 1,200 ml/min.

In life, the situation is more complex but probably an increased cardiac output is achieved mainly by the change in rate, augmented in some circumstances by improved ventricular emptying (Rushmer, 1959). Certainly in man, increases in heart rate alone can enhance the velocity of ventricular contraction (Glick *et al.*, 1965). The variation between Frank–Starling curves represents a change in performance that is probably the result of a change in heart rate augmented to a slight extent by better emptying of the ventricles.

At faster heart rates, the ventricles cannot fill passively so completely as at the slower rates. The intraventricular pressure fails to equal the atrial pressure, and the atrial contraction plays an increasingly important role in ventricular filling (Benchimol, 1969; Mitchell and Shapiro, 1969). The atrium is more compliant than the ventricle and so an increase in atrial pressure produces a greater increase in atrial volume than the same increase in ventricular pressure would produce in ventricular volume. This change in atrial volume means more blood is ejected during atrial systole. The greater atrial emptying enhances ventricular filling and maintains the relationship between right atrial pressure and the ventricular stroke volume. Thus even at fast rates, when atrial contraction is important to ventricular filling, Starling's law remains relevant and the atrial pressure/cardiac output relationship is maintained.

The loss of ventricular compliance ultimately limits the stroke volume so that at maximum exercise when the cardiac output is limited by the ventricular stroke volume, an increase in atrial pressure does not improve the performance (Robinson *et al.,* 1966).

The output of the normal heart can vary widely. If the ability of the heart is expressed as the family of curves relating cardiac output to right atrial pressure, then the appropriate curve is selected mainly by the cardiac rate. The heart rate reflects the influence of sympathetic and parasympathetic activity and which curve is appropriate depends on the work demanded of the heart.

The work done is determined by the cardiac output and the arterial resistance (sometimes called the after-load).

There is a firm relationship between cardiac output and cardiac work, and so performance curves can be expressed in either way. The standard definition of work in physics is:

$$\text{FORCE} \times \text{DISTANCE} = \text{WORK}$$

An alternative expression (*see Figure 3*) is:

$$(\text{FORCE/AREA}) \times \text{DISTANCE} \times \text{AREA} = \text{WORK}$$

The introduction of the area across which the force acts does not alter the equation as area is both a divisor and a multiplier. However, force/area is pressure and moving the area

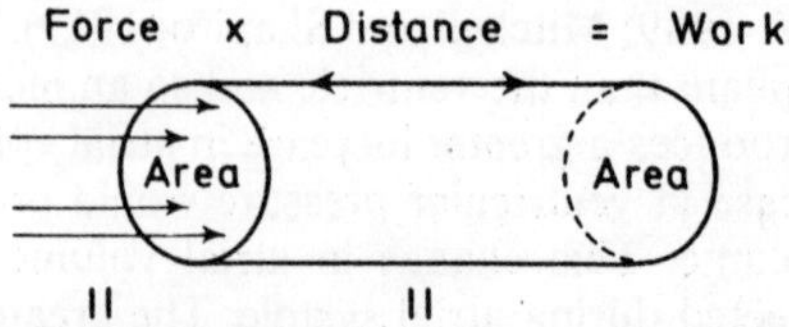

Figure 3.

some distance sweeps out a volume. Thus the work done can also be expressed as:

$$\text{PRESSURE} \times \text{VOLUME} = \text{WORK}$$

If we consider the useful work done per minute as the power of the heart. we have:

$$\underset{\text{(arterial pressure)}}{\text{PRESSURE}} \times \underset{\text{(cardiac output)}}{\text{VOLUME per min}} = \underset{\text{(power of the heart)}}{\text{WORK per min}}$$

Thus performance curves which are expressed in units of cardiac work are referring to the power of the heart. If the arterial pressure is steady then the cardiac power alters with the output, and by assuming a steady arterial pressure we can express the cardiac performance curve simply in terms of cardiac output. In practice the output requirement dominates the performance curve but changes in arterial peripheral resistance do alter the work of the heart. Unless the performance curve of the heart changes, the cardiac output will be altered inversely as the change in resistance. However the normal left ventricle is influenced indirectly by stabilizing mechanisms such as the baroreceptors which make it less sensitive than it would be otherwise to increases in arterial resistance. Only a small decline in output occurs with increased arterial resistance (Guyton *et al.*, 1959; *Figure 4*); that is, the normal left ventricle increases its effective work. Conversely, a lower resistance only slightly alters the performance curve and increases the cardiac output. However, if the ventricle is so badly damaged by disease that its maximal performance curve is low, a useful improvement in cardiac output may be achieved by deliberate vasodilatation. The arterial pressure is lowered as much as is compatible with adequate perfusion and so the greatest cardiac output occurs with the least resistance and there is no increase in work. When cardiac work is limited, the lowest resistance achieves the best flow, for it is flow which provides the vital tissue oxygenation. Careful vasodilatation has been successful in selected patients with severe cardiac failure (Bradley, 1965) and an improved cardiac output with a slight reduction in ventricular filling pressure has been observed (Majid, Sharma and Taylor, 1971).

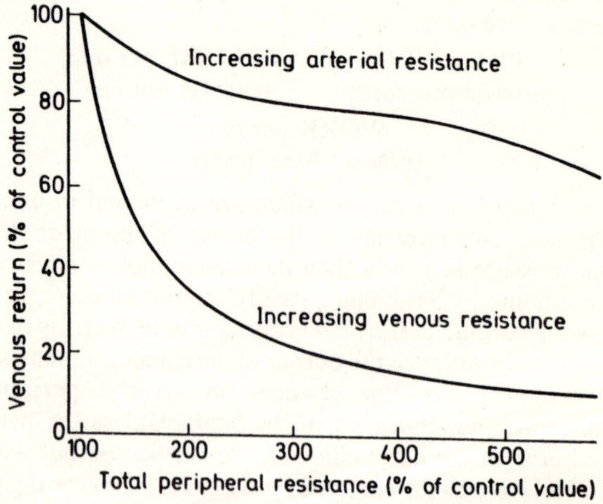

Figure 4. Diagram showing the relative importance of arterial and venous resistance to venous return. As venous return and cardiac output remain equal, this also expresses the effect on the cardiac output. Altering the arterial resistance by a factor of 5, reduces output by about 25 per cent. In contrast, a 5-fold increase in venous resistance reduces flow to about one-eighth of the control value

(Modified from Guyton *et al.* (1959), by courtesy of the authors and the Editors, American Journal of Physiology)

The upper cardiac performance curve can be reduced by heart disease and in this circumstance the same increase in right atrial pressure produces a smaller increase in cardiac output (compare higher and lower performance curves, *Figure 2*). The lower performance curve is probably related to an increased volume remaining in the ventricle at the end of systole. Conversely, increases in the performance of the normal heart (upper curve, *Figure 2*) are produced by sympathetic activity, mainly by an increase in pulse rate. The way in which this happens can be seen clearly by observing the totally denervated heart in man after cardiac transplantation. In these patients exercise can, by increased atrial filling, cause an increase in output without a rise in pulse rate (Campeau *et al.,* 1970). The elevation to a higher performance curve with increase in pulse rate only occurs later, some minutes after the start of exercise, when the adrenaline and noradrenaline which have been released into the circulation have had time to reach the heart (Leachman *et al.,* 1969 a, b; 1971). Ventricular performance curves are a physiological way of estimating the cardiac function, and measurements over several heart rates give a good overall assessment. This indicates how well the heart can meet the demands made on it. Increasing arterial resistance (Ross and Braunwald, 1964) and rate pacing (Parker, Khaja and Case, 1970) have both been used as variables against which changes in left ventricular filling pressure are measured to estimate the performance curve of the left ventricle.

The compliance or ease of ventricular filling is an extremely important factor. It is usually measured as the increase in stroke volume per unit filling pressure. In abnormal hearts, the ventricular compliance may be less than one-third of that found in normal hearts (Parker, Khaja and Case, 1970). Estimates of the performance curve by means of slight increases in filling pressure are helpful in deciding the prognosis after acute myocardial infarction (Bradley, Jenkins and Branthwaite, 1970; Russell *et al.*, 1970). A flat performance curve is associated with a high mortality (Mantle *et al.,* 1973). Cardiac function curves have also been calculated during surgery (Taylor, 1972), and an attempt has been made to use left ventricular function curves as part of a computed index for predicting operative survival of patients with cirrhosis and portal hypertension (Siegel and Williams, 1969).

An estimate of the cardiac performance curve has also been claimed to provide a useful guide as to how well the elderly patient will withstand surgery (Gudwin *et al.,* 1967; Lewin *et al.,* 1971). Two points should be noted. The pulse rate indicates the level of sympathetic enhancement. Generally this level is high in shock but not maximal (Carey *et al.*, 1969). When this level is set, it determines the upper limit for the output of the heart. However, the actual output is determined also by the right atrial pressure, and so it is important to know what factors affect the right atrial pressure.

The venous return

The pressure in the right atrium is the end pressure for blood returning to the right atrium and is the 'vis a fronte' for the venous return. As the venous return is an example of a fluid flowing through closed tubes, this return is governed by physical factors some of which cannot be altered by the regulating systems of the body. These physical factors can be illustrated by a hydraulic model.

If a tank of water has a pipe at the bottom (*Figure 5a*), the outflow through this pipe is governed by simple laws. The simplest is that the flow (Q) is directly related to the pressure at the bottom of the holding tank, so that increasing the height (H) of water in the tank increases the flow in proportion. This is expressed graphically as a straight line (*Figure 5b*) and mathematically as $Q = kH$ where k is a constant related to the resistance of the pipe. If we alter the size of the outflow pipe, we change the flow for a given height of water; however, the relationship between flow and the height of water is still a straight line. Thus we have a family of straight lines (*Figure 5b*). The slope of each line expresses the ease of flow through that particular pipe. In other words, the reciprocal of the slope is an expression of the resistance to flow; thus the flatter the straight line the greater is the resistance.

Similarly we can consider the outflow pipe. The flow increases with the pressure difference between the two ends of the pipe (ΔP). It also increases as the fourth power of the radius of the pipe, so that doubling the width of the pipe increases flow to sixteen times its previous rate. Two things reduce flow, an increase in the viscosity of the liquid and an increase in the length of the pipe. Thus a plot of the radius (r) against flow (Q) gives a fourth power curve in which flow increases rapidly as the width increases; a 19 per cent increase doubles the flow (*Figure 5c*). Since, as mentioned above, the flow in a given pipe increases with the pressure gradient which is the head of water in the tank, we have again a family of curves (*Figure 5c*); the slope increases with the head of

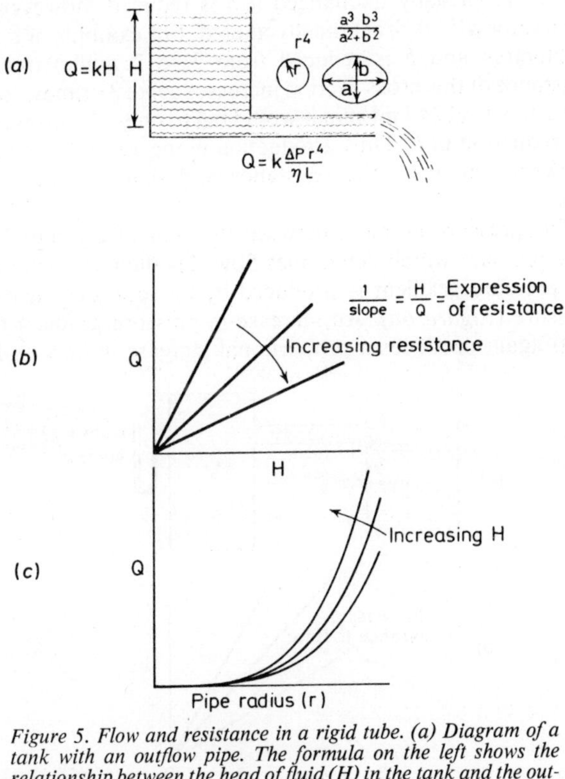

Figure 5. Flow and resistance in a rigid tube. (a) Diagram of a tank with an outflow pipe. The formula on the left shows the relationship between the head of fluid (H) in the tank and the outflow (Q). This is shown graphically in (b). The formula at the bottom of (a) shows the relationship between the pipe parameters and the outflow (Poiseuille's equation). (c) The relationship between the pipe radius (r) and the outflow

(Formula from Alexander, 1963)

pressure. If the pipe has an elliptical rather than a circular cross-section, the factor r^4 must be modified and becomes:

$$\frac{a^3b^3}{a^2 + b^2} \text{ (see Figure 5a)}$$

where a and b are the axes of the cross-section. This has important consequences: if b is much less than a, the denominator $a^2 + b^2$ is virtually unchanged if b is reduced; however, the numerator a^3b^3 is dramatically altered. For example, if a is 10 millimetres and b is reduced from 3 to 2 millimetres, the resistance of this cross-section increases some $3\frac{1}{2}$ times, so that if the flow was 247 ml/min it would fall to only 77 ml/min with the reduction in b. Thus a reduction in the smaller dimension markedly increases the resistance and sharply reduces the flow.

The pressure gradient between the ends of the pipe is the only pressure which determines flow. The flow is unaltered if the pressure gradient is produced by an equivalent negative pressure (*Figure 6a*). An increase in pressure gradient (suction) again produces a proportional increase in flow and the

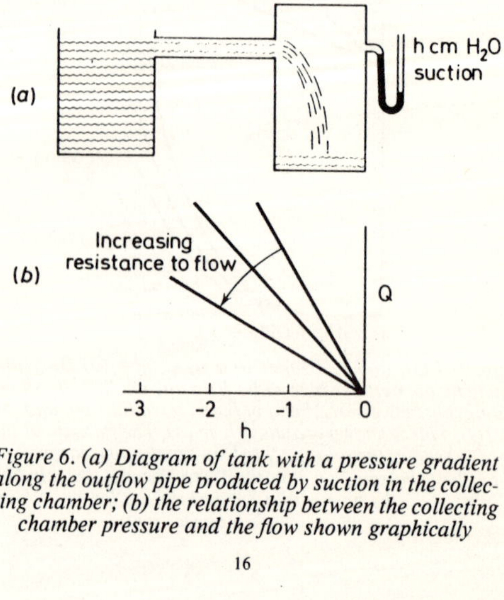

Figure 6. (a) Diagram of tank with a pressure gradient along the outflow pipe produced by suction in the collecting chamber; (b) the relationship between the collecting chamber pressure and the flow shown graphically

plot of flow (Q) against suction (h) is linear. The slope of the graph of pressure and flow still expresses the ease of flow or, inversely, the resistance (*Figure 6b*), as before.

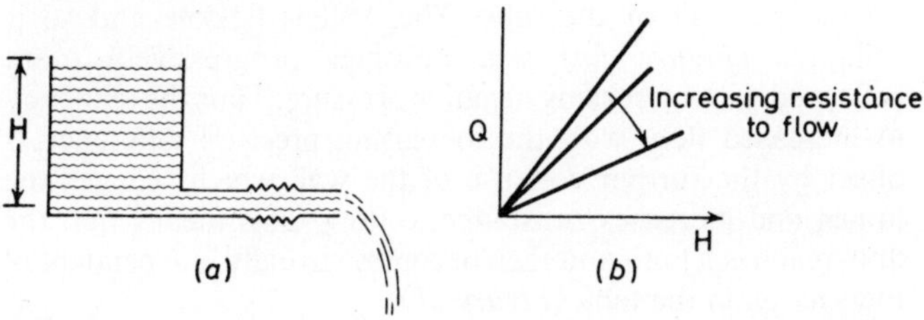

Figure 7. Flow and resistance in a pliable tube. This diagram is similar to Figure 4(a and b) but with a pliable outflow pipe. The head of fluid still has a proportional effect on the outflow

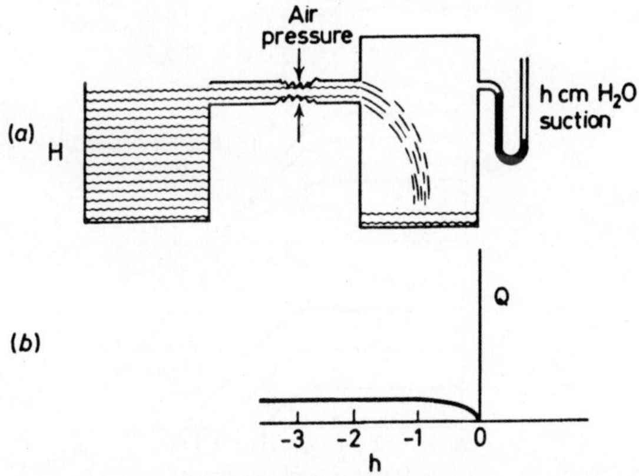

Figure 8. (a) Diagram of flow through a pliable pipe with suction in the collecting tank. Collapse of the pipe increases resistance and limits flow; (b) graphical representation of the flow with increasing suction in the collecting tank

Some further modification is necessary before we have a model which can satisfactorily mimic the situation in the veins. If we alter the pipe by making it flexible, there is still a linear relationship between the flow and the height of water (*Figure 7*). If, however, we now make the pressure gradient with suction the relationship between the flow and the pressure gradient is different. The negative pressure produces a pressure gradient across the wall of the tube. The wall is flexible and so it collapses (*Figure 8a*) and becomes progressively more collapsed with increasing negative pressure. Thus the tendency to increased flow with the increasing pressure difference is offset by the further collapse of the wall which reduces the lumen and increases resistance to flow. This means that the flow reaches a limit and then becomes virtually independent of the suction in the tank (*Figure 8b*).

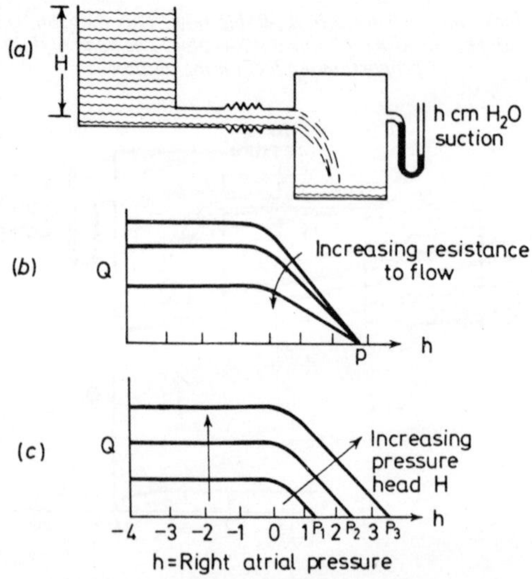

Figure 9. (a) Diagram of combined feed and collecting tanks with a pliable pipe. (b) Graph of flow from changing pressure in the collecting tank. The three curves are for three diameters of pipe. P is the pressure where there is no flow. (c) Graph of flow from changing pressure in the collecting tank. The three curves are for three different heads of pressure in the feed tank: as the pressure increases the point of no flow also increases (P_1, P_2 and P_3)

If a holding tank of water is linked to a suction tank by a pliable tube, there is a combined effect (*Figure 9a*). When the initial pressure in the 'suction' tank is positive and equal to the head of pressure in the holding tank, there is no pressure gradient along the pipe: the pressure in the suction tank is now a measure of the head of pressure in the holding tank. As the pressure in the suction tank is reduced, the flow increases until the pressure becomes negative and the wall of the pliable tube begins to collapse. At this pressure the flow no longer increases and any increase in pressure difference by increasing suction only collapses the tube further and increases the resistance to flow. The increased resistance offsets the increase in pressure gradient along the tube that would otherwise increase flow.

A diagram of suction (*h*) and flow (*Q*) is shown in *Figure 9b*. The pressure at which there is no flow along the tube (at *P*) is determined only by the head of pressure in the holding tank. As pressure alters in *Figure 9c*, so does the point of no flow at successively 1.4, 2.5 and 3.6 cm H_2O pressure. Changing the head of pressure also alters the limit of flow. The slope of the line from the point of no flow is a reciprocal function of the resistance of the tube (*Figure 9b* and *c*). A flatter slope indicates a greater resistance to flow. The limit of flow is altered by a change in resistance or a change in the head of pressure (*H*). The region of inflexion on the graph is the pressure at which collapse begins to occur. The collapse is at the same negative pressure in all circumstances because the major cause is atmospheric pressure and this is unaltered.

This model can provide insight into the working of the venous system. The head of pressure in the holding tank is analogous to the venous capillary pressure at the tissue level, the 'vis a tergo' or the mean systemic pressure. The pliable tube represents the veins and the suction tank the right atrium. Animal studies have demonstrated the aptness of this model (Guyton *et al.*, 1957). The mean systemic pressure is defined as the pressure in the systemic circulation under the existing conditions of vessels and blood volume but with zero flow. This is closely linked to the pressure driving the blood back to the heart.

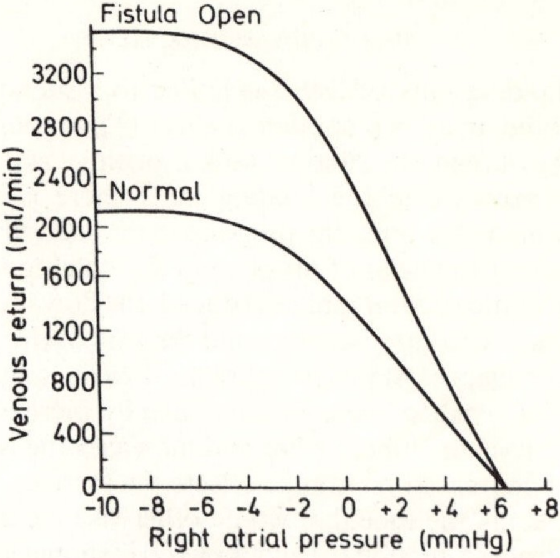

Figure 10. Graph of venous return at various right atrial pressures with and without a large fistula. The region of zero flow is unchanged (6.5 mmHg) and the region of inflexion is also the same (–6 to 0 mmHg)

(Modified from Guyton and Sagawa (1961), by courtesy of the authors and the Editors, American Journal of Physiology)

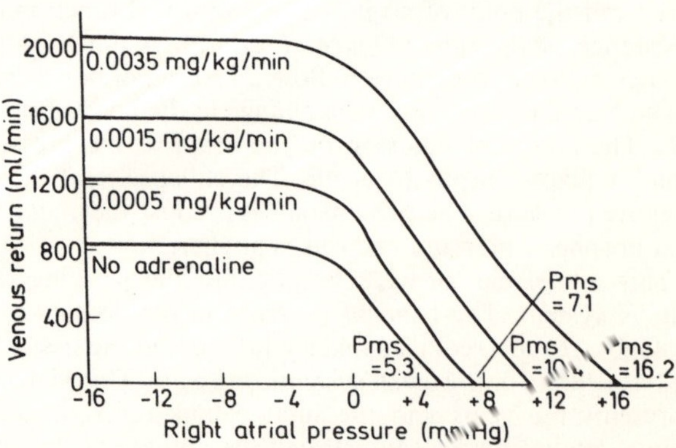

Figure 11. Effect of adrenaline on dogs under total spinal anaesthesia to block all autonomic reflexes. Venous return is increased with increasing doses of adrenaline. Pms is mean systemic circulatory pressure which also increases but in a parallel manner. The region of inflexion remains unaltered (–4 to +2 mmHg)

(Modified from Guyton *et al.* (1958a), by courtesy of the authors and the Editors, American Journal of Physiology)

If an arteriovenous fistula is opened the venous resistance is reduced (Guyton and Sagawa, 1961; *Figure 10*) and it is this that gives the improved flow for the same pressure gradient (cf. *Figure 9b*). Note that the region of inflexion—the pressure where the flow of blood becomes limited—is unchanged; the decrease in resistance improves flow but the inflexion occurs over the same range of right atrial pressures. Similarly, in dogs

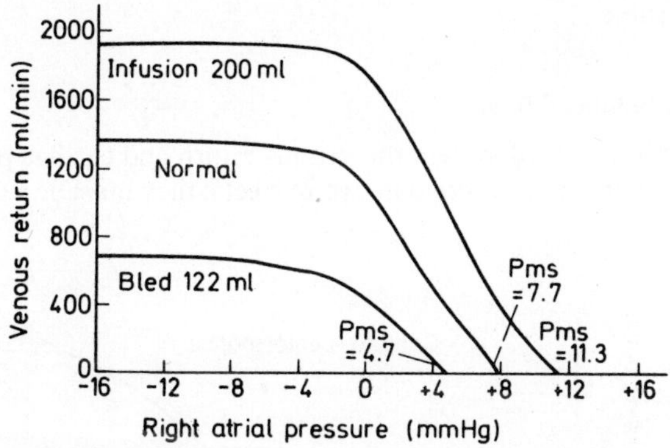

Figure 12. Effect of changing blood volume in dogs under total spinal anaesthesia. Venous return increases with increasing volume. The mean systemic pressure also increases. The slopes of the venous return at positive right atrial pressures become steeper as volume increases (lower venous resistance). The region of inflexion in all three curves is the same
(Modified from Guyton *et al.* (1958b), by courtesy of the authors and the Editors, American Journal of Physiology)

which have a total spinal anaesthetic to abolish all sympathetic activity, an increase in venous tone, or in the mean systemic pressure, produces an increase in venous return for a given right atrial pressure, with no change in the venous resistance, as illustrated by the unchanged initial slope in *Figure 11* (Guyton *et al.*, 1958a). Again, the region of inflexion is unaffected and remains at the same right atrial pressure (cf. *Figure 9c*).

A change in blood volume alters the vessel size, which changes the venous resistance and the vessel tone, which reflects the mean systemic pressure of the system. Thus if dogs which have a total block of sympathetic activity are bled, they show a lower mean systemic pressure and a flatter initial slope for their venous return than do dogs with a normal blood volume. Similarly, dogs which are infused with extra blood show the reverse effects on venous tone and resistance (Guyton *et al.*, 1958b; *Figure 12*). However, despite all these changes the right atrial pressures at the region of inflexion are the same.

The balanced flow

In this closed system the venous return and cardiac performance must correspond in two respects: they must be working

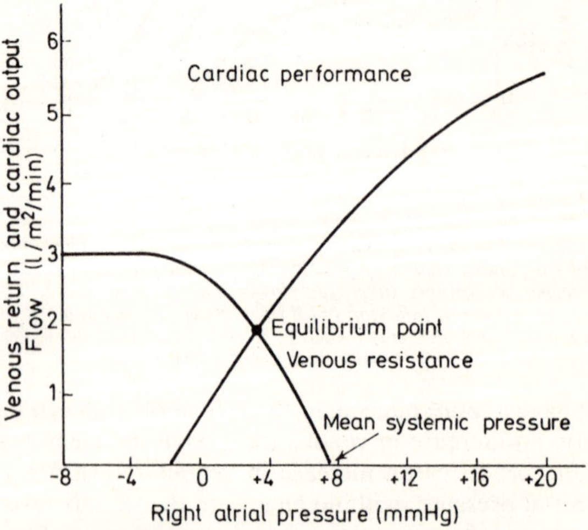

Figure 13. Diagram of venous return and cardiac output as they are each affected by right atrial pressure. The venous return curve depends on the mean systemic pressure and venous resistance. The cardiac curve depends on the autonomic state and the condition of the ventricular muscle. At only one value of right atrial pressure do the venous return and cardiac output correspond

at the same flow—that is, the blood returned must be pumped on, and this must be done at the same right atrial pressure (*Figure 13*). At any one time, there can be only one right atrial pressure and one flow where the prevailing venous return and prevailing cardiac output are in equilibrium. This is illustrated by the point at which the performance curve and the venous return curve cross in *Figure 13*.

If the venous tone rises, the mean systemic pressure rises and the venous performance curve must rise also. The higher venous curve means that the right atrial pressure rises and the equilibrium point is now at a greater cardiac output. The output can fall again only if the cardiac performance curve is depressed and the upper limit of output reduced.

EXAMPLES OF NORMAL REGULATION

Sympathetic Effects

Increased sympathetic activity affects both the heart and the venous system. The effect on the heart is that the cardiac performance curve becomes more sensitive to changes in the pressure in the right atrium and the upper limit for the cardiac output is set higher (*Figure 14*). This increased sympathetic activity is associated with a rise in pulse rate. An elevated cardiac performance alone would reduce the right atrial pressure but have only a modest effect in improving output if the venous return curve remained the same (*see* open circle at A, *Figure 14*). However, sympathetic activity also increases venous tone which elevates the venous curve and achieves a greater return for the same right atrial pressure (Banet and Guyton, 1971). The combined effect of the sympathetic activity in elevating venous tone and cardiac performance achieves an increased cardiac output with little or no change in right atrial pressure.

The Cardiovascular Response to Exercise

During exercise sympathetic activity has a large effect on venous return and cardiac performance. In addition, many small vessels open up, particularly in the active muscles, and the physiological effect of this dilatation of small vessels is like that of a fistula. As previously discussed, a fistula elevates the

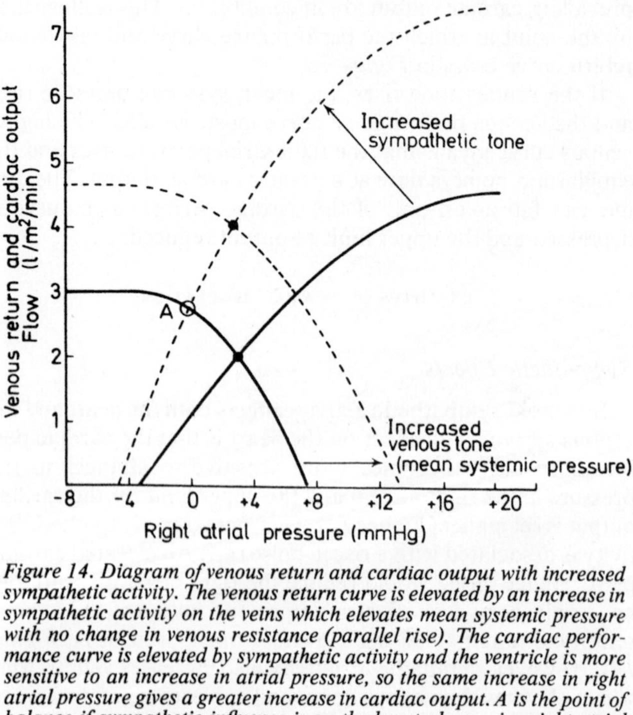

Figure 14. Diagram of venous return and cardiac output with increased sympathetic activity. The venous return curve is elevated by an increase in sympathetic activity on the veins which elevates mean systemic pressure with no change in venous resistance (parallel rise). The cardiac performance curve is elevated by sympathetic activity and the ventricle is more sensitive to an increase in atrial pressure, so the same increase in right atrial pressure gives a greater increase in cardiac output. A is the point of balance if sympathetic influence is on the heart alone—i.e. right atrial pressure would fall. However, the change in the venous return curve tends to elevate the right atrial pressure which means the overall effect is an increased cardiac output with no change in pressure

venous return curve (*see Figure 10*), the peripheral veins are dilated and the total effect is a lower venous resistance which elevates the venous return curve (*Figure 15*). Again cardiac output is greatly increased with little or no change in right atrial pressure. Under conditions of maximal exercise right

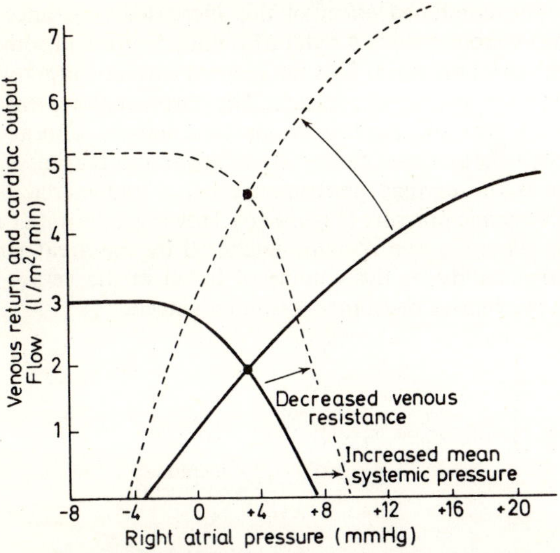

Figure 15. Diagram of venous return and cardiac output during exercise. The increased sympathetic activity elevates the cardiac performance and increases the mean systemic pressure. The venous resistance decreases as more muscle vessels open

atrial pressure may rise, but this does not further improve the output of a normal heart (Robinson *et al.,* 1966).

EXAMPLES OF ACUTE PATHOLOGICAL UPSET

Blood Loss

The immediate effect of an acute loss of blood is felt in the venous system. The circulating blood volume is reduced and much of this loss is distributed in the venous side of the circulation. The lower capacity of the venous system is accompanied by a lower venous tone and the resistance to flow in the veins is increased because the vessels are narrowed (*Figure 16*). Brobmann *et al.* (1971) suggest that a 30 per cent haemorrhage increases the resistance of the larger veins by almost 260 per cent. The combined effect of this increased resistance and reduced venous tone is a reduced venous return and some fall in right atrial pressure. This fall reduces cardiac output which causes a lower arterial pressure. The baroreceptors sense the lower pressure and increase sympathetic activity. This activity reduces venous capacitance (Hainsworth and Karim, 1974), improves the cardiac performance curve and increases the mean systemic pressure (*Figure 16*). However, the initial slope of the venous curve remains unaltered by the greater sympathetic activity as the volume of blood in the veins—and hence the venous resistance—is not changed.

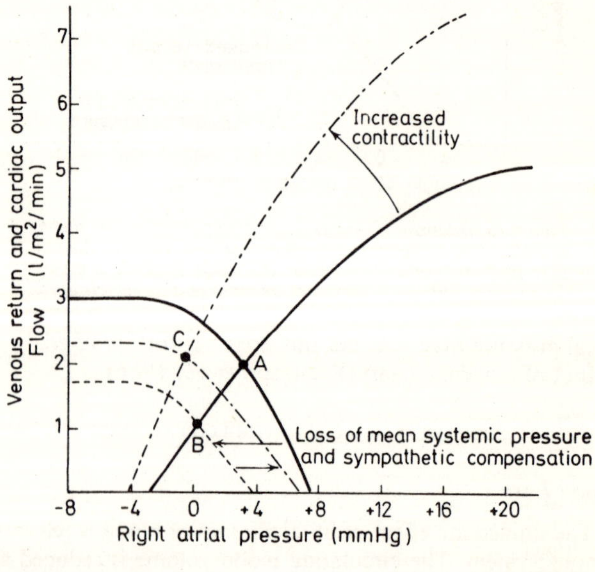

Figure 16. Diagram of venous return and cardiac output after an acute loss of blood. The normal curves are given as continuous lines and the normal flow/pressure point is marked at A. The cardiac performance is elevated by the sympathetic response which also elevates the mean systemic pressure (C). If the sympathetic response is absent, the cardiac output and venous return are markedly reduced (lower dot B). The reduced blood volume means an increased venous resistance (and a flatter slope for the venous return curve)

The normal right atrial pressure in man is about 6 mmHg (Robson, 1968; *see* discussion later however) which is positive of the inflexion in the venous return curve. Thus the fall in right atrial or central venous pressure that occurs with blood loss is due partly to the changes in the venous return curve caused by loss of venous tone and the increase in venous resistance and partly to the improved cardiac performance resulting from the increased sympathetic activity.

Three special situations must be considered. First, if the sympathetic response to the loss of blood is reduced or absent, the fall in right atrial pressure is less for the same volume of blood loss and the fall in cardiac output will be greater. Here, changes in the venous return curve occur (to B, *Figure 16*) but no sympathetic elevation in mean systemic pressure follows, nor is the cardiac performance curve elevated. Secondly, if the right atrial pressure is already less than the inflexion region of the venous return curve, any increase in sympathetic stimulation to the heart cannot alter the cardiac output which is now limited by the venous return. However, a further fall in right atrial pressure may be seen. Thus a fall in right atrial pressure following increased sympathetic stimulation (such as an isoprenaline infusion would produce) indicates a need to improve the venous return curve but does not necessarily indicate that the sympathetic stimulation has achieved an increase in cardiac output. Finally, further bleeding may cause only a slight fall in right atrial pressure once the sympathetic activity is maximal, although a large fall in cardiac output can occur. This is because the sympathetic activity elevates the cardiac performance curve. The heart is more sensitive to changes in right atrial pressure so that a decrease in atrial pressure causes a greater fall in cardiac output. Thus the volume of blood lost cannot be related directly to the amount of change in pressure in the right atrium if the level of sympathetic activity is changing.

Myocardial Infarction

Infarction of the myocardium from any cause means that there is a loss of functioning myocardium. About 95 per cent of all infarcts involve the left ventricle (Wartman and Kellerstein, 1948), so left ventricular function is almost always affected. This loss of myocardium impairs ventricular emptying and reduces the cardiac performance. Less functioning myocardium means that for the same venous return curve, cardiac output is lower and pressure in the atrium is higher

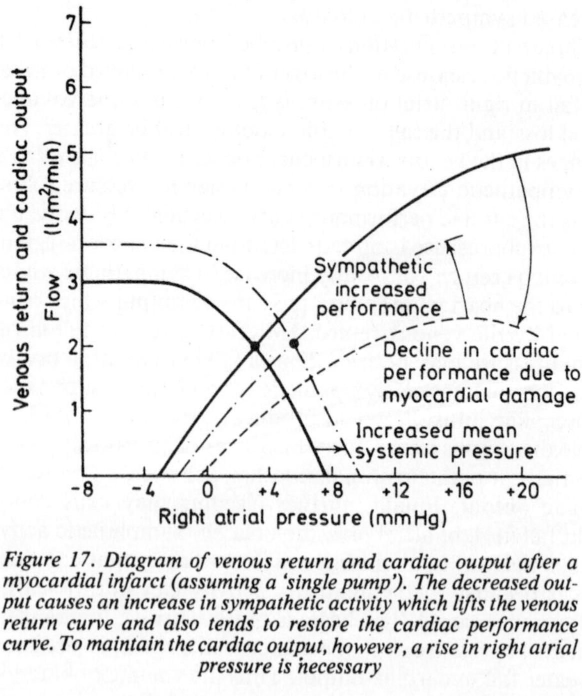

Figure 17. Diagram of venous return and cardiac output after a myocardial infarct (assuming a 'single pump'). The decreased output causes an increase in sympathetic activity which lifts the venous return curve and also tends to restore the cardiac performance curve. To maintain the cardiac output, however, a rise in right atrial pressure is necessary

(*Figure 17*). The compensatory mechanisms enhance sympathetic activity and both cardiac performance and venous tone are thereby increased. A sympathetic increase in venous tone plays a significant role in raising the venous return curve and the right atrial pressure. A very high left atrial pressure may produce pulmonary venous engorgement and raise the pulmonary arterial pressure. This increases the work of the right heart and may elevate right atrial pressure further. A greatly increased right atrial pressure indicates that there is a marked increase in venous tone and it is probable that the myocardium is badly damaged: left atrial pressure is probably also elevated. Such patients are recognized as having a poor prognosis (Collins *et al.*, 1971).

The oxygen requirement of the body must be met during the acute deficiency in cardiac performance and the oxygen transport via the cardiovascular system must continue in order to answer this demand. A number of factors affect oxygen transport (Nunn and Freeman, 1964) but in this acute situation either the cardiac output must be maintained or oxygen extraction must be increased to maintain an adequate supply to the tissues. If the reserve oxygen-carrying capacity cannot cover the deficit in cardiac output, the patient is likely to die. This is why, in practice, right atrial oxygen saturations have been found to correlate well with the patient's condition (Ramo *et al.,* 1970). Although Cournand and his co-workers (1943), in their classic work on shock, found that a quiet shocked patient has a lower oxygen consumption, there is a strict limit to how much consumption can be reduced.

This problem of deficient oxygenation has been explored and discussed by Crowell (1970). Anaerobic metabolism can cover a very brief oxygen debt such as may occur during strenuous exercise, but the lactic acid from this metabolism must eventually be metabolized with oxygen. A serious sign of inadequate oxygen transport is a metabolic acidosis which recurs after correction because the metabolic needs of the body can only be fully met with a supplement of anaerobic metabolism.

Pulmonary Oedema

Pulmonary oedema occurs when the mechanical and osmotic pressures in the alveolar capillaries are no longer in equilibrium. Acute pulmonary oedema is usually caused by a rise in pressure within the alveolar capillaries which is the result of a sudden increase in left atrial pressure. The simple 'single pump' model can no longer adequately simulate the situation and we must consider a more complex model with a right and left heart and a pulmonary circulation in between to mimic these effects realistically.

Although right and left ventricular outputs are controlled by similar factors, the performance curve for each ventricle is

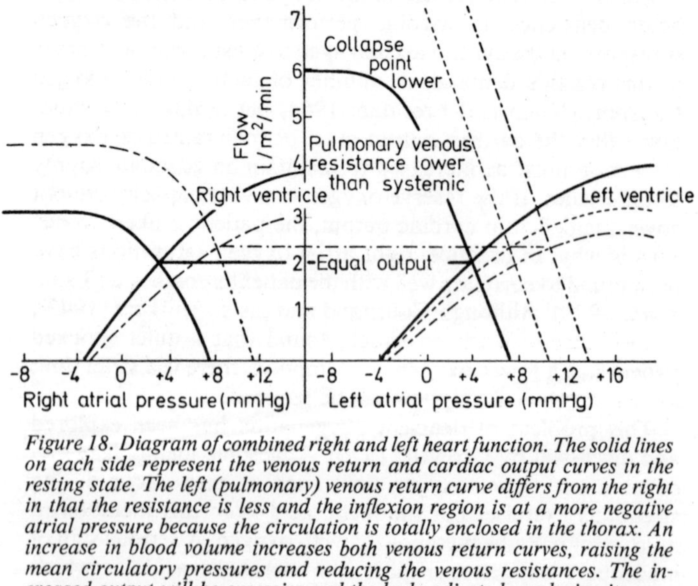

Figure 18. Diagram of combined right and left heart function. The solid lines on each side represent the venous return and cardiac output curves in the resting state. The left (pulmonary) venous return curve differs from the right in that the resistance is less and the inflexion region is at a more negative atrial pressure because the circulation is totally enclosed in the thorax. An increase in blood volume increases both venous return curves, raising the mean circulatory pressures and reducing the venous resistances. The increased output will be excessive and the body adjusts by reducing its sympathetic activity, thus depressing the cardiac performance curve. This is represented by the broken lines. The rise in left atrial pressure and the amount of left ventricular depression depend upon the pulmonary compliance

different (*Figure 18*). This is because the muscle of the left ventricular wall is thicker than the muscle of the right so the left ventricle is less compliant. An increase in left atrial pressure produces a smaller increase in stroke volume (Bishop and Stone, 1967).

The pulmonary venous return curve also differs from the systemic venous return curve. It has a steeper initial slope because the pulmonary venous resistance is lower than the systemic venous resistance. Also, the inflexion region of the pulmonary venous return curve is at a more negative pressure because the pulmonary circulation is completely within the chest and the collapse of the pulmonary veins is caused by the intrathoracic pressure which is sub-atmospheric. Pulmonary veins are also very pliable and an increase in left atrial pressure markedly decreases pulmonary venous resistance (Kuramito and Rodbards, 1962). The mean pulmonary vascular pressure is normally about the same as the mean systemic pressure (Guyton, 1963) at +7 mmHg, or maybe slightly higher but the change in mean pulmonary pressure as expressed by the left atrial pressure tends to exceed the change in mean systemic or right atrial pressure for a given flow (Freitas *et al.,* 1965; Moss *et al.,* 1969). This is the clinical result of the difference in compliance of the ventricles.

An increased fluid load can produce pulmonary oedema as additional fluid produces a greater rise in left than in right atrial pressure: this can occur even in a normal heart. Once the increase in blood volume exceeds 17 per cent there is a consistent rise in cardiac output (Thomasson, 1959). A failing left ventricle may have an extremely poor cardiac performance curve so that the cardiac output can be maintained only by the left atrial pressure rising above the level at which pulmonary oedema is likely to occur. This level is considered to be about 24 mmHg (Guyton and Lindsey, 1959) but is affected by the level of plasma protein (Gaar *et al.,* 1967; Gutierrez *et al.,* 1970). In clinical practice pulmonary oedema usually occurs with a left atrial pressure of 30 mmHg or higher (Wood, 1968).

Pulmonary oedema may also occur suddenly after myocardial damage such as an infarct. The damaged myocardium causes the left ventricular curve to be depressed and the difference in performance between the right and left ventricles is exaggerated. The left atrial pressure needed to maintain cardiac output is higher and greater changes in atrial pressure are needed to achieve changes in output. The left ventricle may be so badly damaged that even the normal resting output requires an excessive left atrial pressure. Such myocardial depression or damage may produce pulmonary oedema without a rise in right atrial pressure (Simmons *et al.,* 1969a). Certainly the right atrial or central venous pressure is no more than a guide to left atrial pressure. The two may be related only statistically even with a normal myocardium (Moss *et al.,* 1969). However, if a good baseline for the central venous pressure can be established and myocardial function is normal, a rise will effectively warn of impending pulmonary oedema (Andersen and Klebe, 1968b).

The management of acute pulmonary oedema in over-load or myocardial failure must be directed at reducing left atrial pressure. This means reducing the mean pulmonary vascular pressure by phlebotomy or sympathetic blockade (Dykes and Fuller, 1969; Gould *et al.,* 1970), or improving cardiac performance by cardiotonic drugs. Digoxin would seem to be the drug of choice (Visscher *et al.,* 1956) and would not alter mean systemic or pulmonary pressures. Adrenaline would appear to be inappropriate as it has been shown to produce pulmonary oedema in some species (Visscher *et al.,* 1956). Presumably the cardiotonic effect of adrenaline is outweighed by its vascular effects, particularly those effects which increase the mean venous pressure.

Chronic heart disease

In a previously normal heart, the physiological changes in acute illness are predictable. Often a good estimate of the severity of the acute disease and also of the effectiveness of treatment can be obtained by matching the expected values of cardiovascular parameters against the values actually observed. Thus, a useful assessment of the cardiovascular state is possible, by comparing the pulse rate, blood pressure, central venous pressure, and perfusion rate (e.g., as estimated crudely by capillary refilling and urinary output) with what they should be. In this way the severity of myocardial infarction or, say, haemorrhagic shock can be judged and logical steps taken to improve the patient's condition.

Chronic heart disease limits the ability of the heart to respond and may modify the observed values of some of the cardiac measurements. For example, chronic pulmonary hypertension may cause an elevated right atrial pressure. During haemorrhage the right atrial pressure will fall to normal levels, but then it is too low and volume replacement is necessary. A similar situation may occur in congestive cardiac failure in which venous tone may already be increased fourfold (Sharpey-Schafer, 1963). Mitral valve disease places a severe and abnormal load on the pulmonary vasculature which becomes thickened. The usually close relationship between right and left atrial pressure may be lost so that with catecholamine stimulation, with changes in heart rate or with volume loading, the pressure changes in the right and left atria are no longer correlated.

These examples demonstrate that when there is serious chronic heart disease as many cardiovascular factors as possible should be independently monitored. Generally the most important additional measurement to those usually made, is that of left atrial pressure.

The longer view

This discussion has centred on the acute effects, but there are many other changes which could have a long-term influence on both venous return and cardiac performance. For example, we can examine the situation after blood loss. Some influences will counteract the loss. A reduced cardiac output reduces renal flow (Stone and Stahl, 1970) which helps to maintain the effective blood volume, and a reduced capillary pressure allows a net influx of fluid into the circulation and tends to restore blood volume over a period of hours. Conversely, if haemorrhagic shock persists for a prolonged period—say, more than 10 hours—a complicating myocardial depression may occur (Carey *et al.*, 1967) with the result that fluid replacement alone is no longer adequate (Siegel and Downing, 1970).

II
Central Venous Pressure in Clinical Use

Assessment of Cardiac Output

Even when the physiology and dynamic pathology of the cardiovascular system are understood the practical details of central venous pressure measurement remain to be mastered.

The measurement is not appropriate in every patient but it should be made whenever the cardiovascular dynamics are abnormal. Clinically this may be obvious as pulmonary oedema or, more commonly, as an inadequate cardiac output. Thus an assessment of the adequacy of the cardiac output will often be the first consideration.

If it is decided that the central venous pressure should be measured, then the practical matters of technique and evaluation of the measurements follow.

The most critical transport requirement in the body is that for oxygen. For many tissues an adequate oxygenation is supremely important. It is the oxygen supply that is limited by flow in hypotension (Crowell, 1970) and the consequent enforced reduction in oxidative metabolism may damage some tissues. Many factors affect the need of the tissues for oxygen. Even at rest the individual requirement may be greatly different; from, for example, an abnormal low in myxoedema, to a very high level in fever or during shivering.

Important indicators for assessing the adequacy of cardiac output are found at capillary level. Good capillary filling with a warm pink skin indicates an adequate cardiac output; a pale or blue cold skin suggests poor perfusion and implies that output is inadequate. The function of tissues can also be used in the assessment. If brain perfusion is impaired as shown by a clouded consciousness and poor kidney perfusion is revealed by a low urinary output, it is probable that the cardiac output is

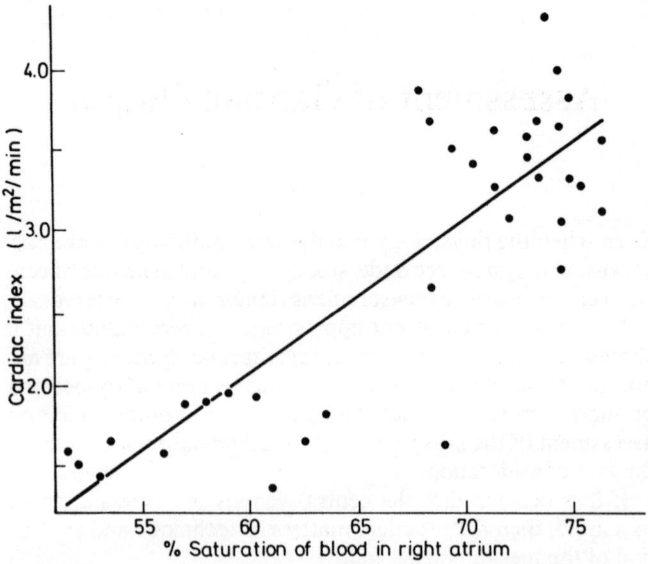

Figure 19. The relationship between oxygen saturation and cardiac output in 36 patients, 13 of whom were considered to be in shock. The output has been standardized as the cardiac index. The correlation coefficient is +0.84 with a regression equation of cardiac index (y) against saturation (x) of $y = 0.0974x - 3.76$

(Drawn from the data of Lee *et al.*, 1972)

inadequate for the patient's requirements (Motsay *et al.*, 1970). When the cardiac output is low, the blood pressure is usually low (below 90/40 mmHg) and the pulse rate high (an indication of increased sympathetic activity in a heart with normal conduction).

A central venous catheter should be introduced if the patient has an inadequate cardiac output. If the catheter is placed in the right atrium, measurement of central venous oxygen content—an index of tissue oxygenation—can provide a further guide to assessment of the general level of perfusion. Even the less sophisticated measurement of oxygen saturation has a good correlation with the cardiac output (*Figure 19*) in shock (Lee, *et al.,* 1972). It has also been found suitable as a guide in patients with myocardial infarction (Goldman *et al.,* 1968) and in severely ill cardiac patients (Scheinman, Brown and Rapaport, 1969).

In normal subjects the relationship between the oxygen saturation of blood from the superior vena cava, right atrium, right ventricle and pulmonary artery is very close (Barrat-Boyes and Wood, 1957). This relationship is less close in low cardiac output states; in particular, a blood sample from the superior vena cava tends to have a higher oxygen saturation than do samples from the other sites (Lee *et al.,* 1972; Scheinman, Brown and Rapaport, 1969). However, from any of these sites changes in saturation have the same implication—that a change in perfusion has occurred.

The Technique of Measurement

Insertion of a central venous catheter

Today most clinicians prefer to avoid the inferior vena cava because of the risk of sepsis in the groin (Bansmer *et al.,* 1958) and because any increase in abdominal pressure makes the readings unreliable (Guyton and Adkins, 1954; *Figure 20*). The increase in abdominal pressure may be caused by disease—for example, a large amount of ascites; or by a normal situation—such as the enlarged uterus of late pregnancy which may elevate the pressure in the inferior vena cava by as

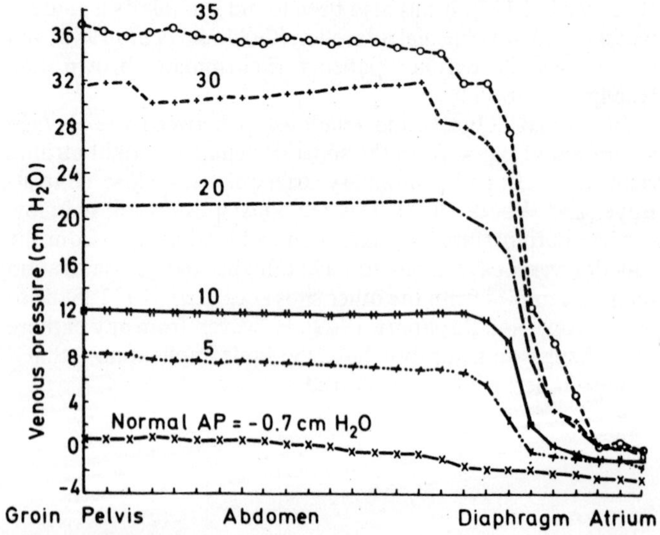

Figure 20. Diagram of pressure measured at various levels in the inferior vena caval system under conditions of raised intra-abdominal pressure (in dogs). The number above each curve is the pressure in the abdomen in cm H_2O. Until the catheter is within the chest the pressure recorded reflects the pressure in the abdomen and not the pressure in the right atrium

(Modified from Guyton and Adkins (1954) by courtesy of the authors and the Editors, American Journal of Physiology)

much as 20 cm H_2O (Kerr, Scott and Samuel, 1964; Colditz, 1970). Often a catheter is passed from the cubital fossa to the superior vena cava or one of its central tributaries, either by a cut-down, Seldinger technique (Seldinger, 1953; Doty, 1969) or a percutaneous stab (Webre and Arens, 1973). Sometimes more direct approaches to a central vein are made (*Figure 21*) either by Aubaniac's (1952) infraclavicular approach to the subclavian vein (Davidson *et al.,* 1963), a supraclavicular subclavian technique (Yoffa, 1965) or a direct approach into the internal jugular vein (English *et al.,* 1969). With any of these techniques the catheter should be radio-opaque or have a radio-opaque line so that the position of the end in the chest may be determined by radiography (Woods *et al.*, 1974).

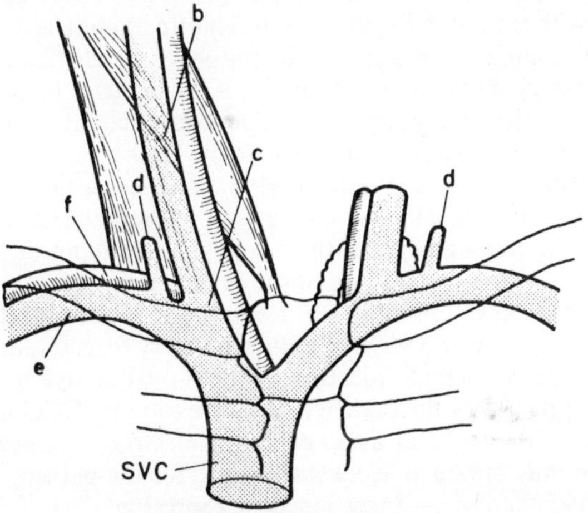

Figure 21. Approaches to the superior vena cava (SVC), b and c indicate percutaneous internal jugular vein cannulations; d indicates the external jugular approach; e and f indicate the infra- and supra-clavicular approaches to the subclavian vein
(Modified from Rushman *et al.*, 1970)

Alternatively a catheter or cannula may be inserted into an external jugular vein to give an approximate value for the central venous pressure (Jones, 1963). The procedure is simple and convenient, particularly during anaesthesia, but generally there is some obstruction to flow and the true central venous pressure will be 1.5–3.5 cm H_2O lower (Ryan and Howland, 1966); the difference may be less, however, with spontaneous respiration (Stoelting, 1973). Provided the chest remains closed, changes in both internal and external jugular venous pressure reflect the changes in pressure at the right atrium in the supine patient under anaesthesia (Briscoe, 1973). However, peripheral limb veins are unsuitable as their pressure does not reliably reflect the central venous pressure nor do changes correspond with changes in central venous pressure (Eustace, 1970).

When the central venous catheter has been positioned correctly, the pressure reading show's a small fluctuation in time with the patient's respiration. This fluctuation is due to the slight change in intrathoracic pressure which occurs with respiratory movements. However, if the catheter is misplaced into the internal jugular vein, respiratory fluctuation may still occur but the reading will be 2–6 cm H_2O too high (Kellner and Smart, 1972). Frequently, a cardiac variation in the pressure reading can also be seen but this may be damped out by a long thin catheter. If there is any doubt about the central position of the catheter its position should be confirmed by a chest radiograph (Gilday and Downs, 1969) or ECG (Hughes and Macgovern, 1959). Confirmation by chest radiograph may require a small injection of radio-opaque dye to outline clearly the tip of the catheter. Confirmation by ECG depends on using the catheter as an exploring electrode—a procedure which may create an electrical hazard for the patient.

Complications.—Insertion of a central venous catheter is not without risks. The subclavian approaches have been responsible for pneumothoraces, haemorrhage, and sepsis (Smith *et al.,* 1965). Sepsis can be reduced by application of antibiotic ointment and daily re-dressing (Moran, Atwood and Rowe, 1965). However, the risk of complication must be considered as particularly high in less experienced hands (Bernard and Stahl, 1971). The approach from the cubital fossa has also had its share of complications: catheter embolism has been reported frequently (Turner and Sommers, 1954) but more unusual problems such as pericardial tamponade have occurred (Thomas *et al.,* 1969; Brandt *et al.,* 1970). English and his coworkers reported 500 cases in their original series of internal jugular vein catheterizations with only one serious complication—a pneumothorax. However, in other hands (Parikh, 1972), this approach has resulted in a Horner's syndrome, presumably caused by damage to the stellate ganglion. Multiple catheterizations may also present a special hazard: one case of knotting has been reported (Swaroop, 1972).

The reference level

The reference level is extremely important when measuring central venous or atrial pressures because these differ only slightly from atmospheric pressure—generally by less than the equivalent of 10 cm of water or saline. (The specific gravity of isotonic saline is 1.005 which in this context is not significantly different from that of water.)

The common methods of measurement all depend on the presence of a column of liquid between the reference point in the right atrium or central vein and the actual pressure-measuring device. The liquid is generally isotonic electrolyte solution and/or blood. As blood has a specific gravity of 1.06 (Diem and Lentner, 1970), the whole column can be regarded as being of the specific gravity of saline with a maximum error of only 6 per cent of the vertical distance by which the blood/saline interface deviates from reference level. Thus if a saline-filled catheter tip is in the superior vena cava 5 cm vertically above the chosen reference point at the mid-right atrium, the recorded pressure will be 0.3 cm H_2O too low. This error is too small to be clinically important—particularly as it will be a consistent error in successive readings. Generally the difficulty of maintaining a level or defining a level in a patient within even 1 cm is great, and so any possible interface error can be ignored. Sometimes the pressure is expressed as millimetres of mercury (abbreviated mmHg) instead of in centimetres of water (cm H_2O). Mercury is 13.6 times more dense than water so the same pressure only supports a mercury column 1/13.6 as high. Thus a reading of 6.8 cm H_2O becomes 0.5 cmHg or more commonly 5 mmHg.

The most important aspects in practice are that the level should be reproduceable and physiologically meaningful. The reproduceability is extremely important because any error in restoring the reference level will appear directly as part of the pressure. Thus an accidental change in the reference level of 2 cm above the previous reference level would appear as a 2 cm H_2O fall in pressure, which would generally be considered significant. It is therefore fundamental to the measurement of central venous pressure that the reference level shall be consistent. With a 4 cm H_2O reading, a variation in the reference level of $\pm$ 0.5 cm H_2O is just acceptable: a wider variation of, say, $\pm$ 1 cm H_2O is probably not, as this would imply that a change in reading from +5 H_2O on one occasion to +3 cm H_2O on the next, might not mean a true change in central venous pressure at all!

Many levels have been used for reference and the subject has been reviewed briefly by DeBrunner and Bühler (1969). The ideal level should not be influenced by body position and this was the aim of the phlebostatic axis of Winsor and Burch (1945) for man—the intersection of a coronal plane at the fourth intercostal space at the sternum. This level corresponds to the posterior part of the atrium (Pedersen and Husby, 1951).

Other attempts have been made to assess venous pressure in a way that would be independent of hydrostatic pressure and thus unaffected by changes in position. For instance, Holt (1940) positioned 10 normal subjects supine and then prone and obtained an average pressure estimate of 10 cm H_2O at the antecubital vein. He did not attempt to find a superficial anatomical reference level, and indeed this would probably have been unwise if we can judge from the results that he obtained, when using a reference level at the midway of the antero-posterior thoracic diameter. The pressure in 7 of his subjects was greater when they were prone than when they were supine but in the other 3 the reverse was the case. These findings cannot be reconciled with a reference level which is a fixed fraction of the transthoracic diameter. Guyton and Greganti (1956) positioned dogs until they found axes in all three directions that showed almost no change in central venous pressure with position. These three axes met at a point just within the tricuspid valve—which is thus the ideal point for a stable reference level. Unfortunately a catheter is in a very

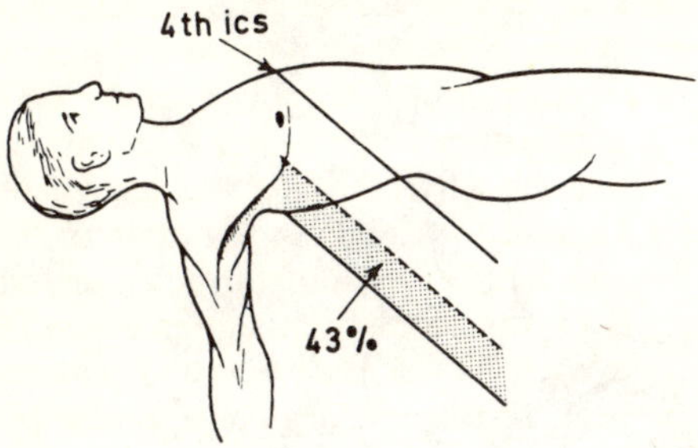

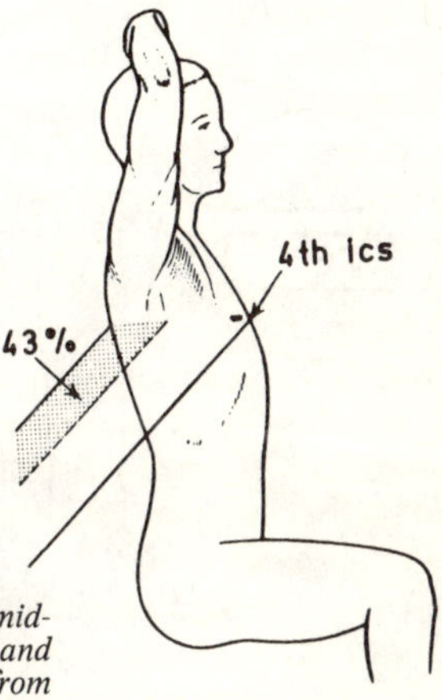

Figure 22. Diagrams of the level of the mid-right atrium as described by Pedersen and Husby, 1951—43 per cent of the distance from the back anterior at the level of the fourth intercostal space anteriorly

unstable position at the tricuspid valve and in practice an estimate of the level of the middle of the right atrium seems as close as we can get to the ideal. A point 43 per cent of the postero-anterior distance from the back to the anterior fourth intercostal space is a fair approximation to the mid-right atrium (Pedersen and Husby, 1951) (*Figure 22*); nevertheless, as a reference level for central venous pressure it is slightly affected by changes in posture and suffers from the individual variation observed by Holt (1940).

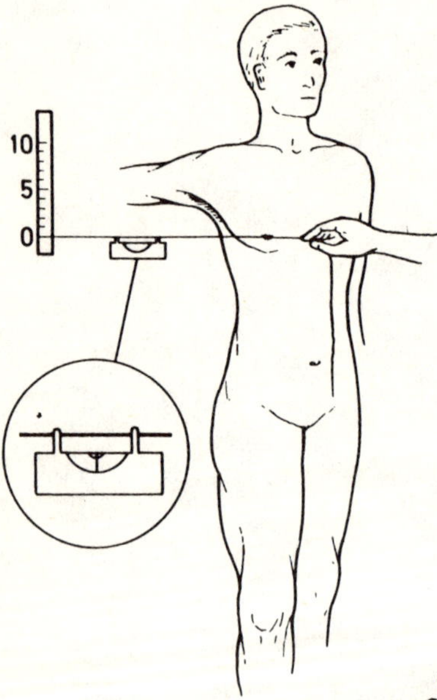

(a)

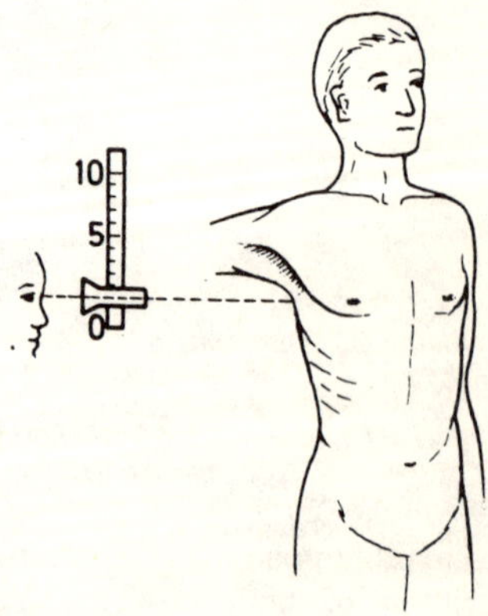

(b)

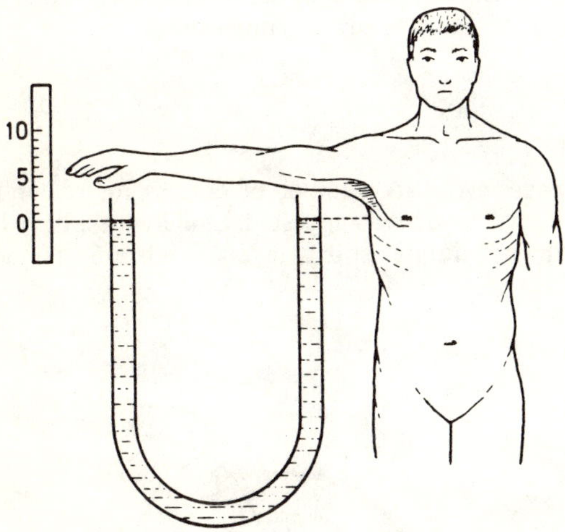

(c)

Figure 23. Diagram of 3 simple devices to assist in determining the reference level: (a) (facing page) shows a small spirit level (inset) on a cord. The line is stretched taut between the zero of the scale and the patient, touching him at the reference level. The spirit level indicates when the line is horizontal and therefore the zero and the chosen reference are at the same level.
(b) (facing page) shows a sight attached to the scale at the zero, which can then set the zero at the reference point. This device does not interfere with the patient but unless care is taken the sighting may not be horizontal and, even worse, repeated sightings may not give the same error.
(c) (above) a manometer sets the true horizontal for the reference level but is cumbersome and messy. The open ends may be joined to form a closed circle, which then avoids any chance of the liquid in the manometer being spilled

Once a reference level has been established, it is important that it should be adhered to. If the mid-right atrial level is chosen as a reference, changes in the patient's position should have only a small effect on the central venous pressure readings.

Apparatus

Reference level.—A number of devices for obtaining the reference level have been suggested. Usually these have been in the form of simple spirit levels, sighting devices, or

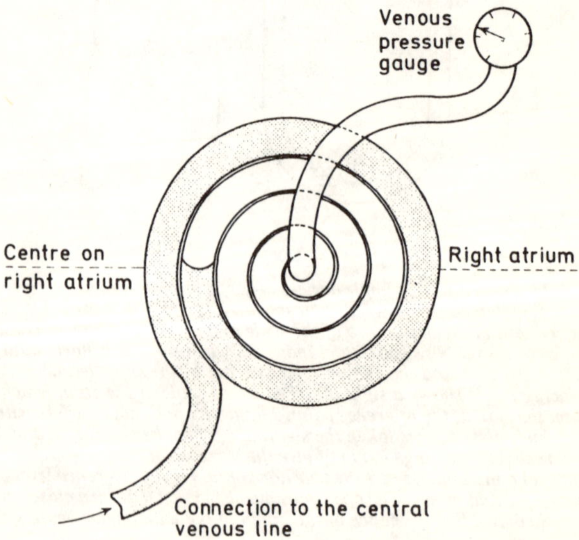

Figure 24. Diagram of the meniscus spiral for stabilizing the reference level in central venous pressure measurement. The spiral tube (about 2 cm in diameter) keeps the meniscus level close to the reference line which is shown here as the right atrium. The pressure on this meniscus then represents the pressure in the right atrium. A small low-volume pressure measuring device is required so that fluctuations in the pressure in the right atrium do not cause the meniscus to go beyond the spiral

(After Latimer, 1971)

manometers (*Figure 23*). With a manometer one meniscus is set at the reference level on the patient's chest and the other meniscus is then used to set the zero for the central venous pressure gauge. An ingenious modification of the usual manometer is a small spiral coil that allows the meniscus to travel along the tube without shifting far from the reference

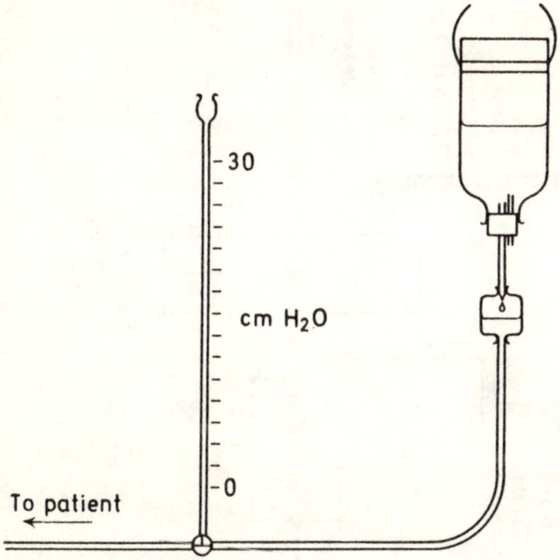

Figure 25. Diagram of a simple fluid manometer for measuring central venous pressure. The zero mark is set to the level of the chosen reference and the tap is turned to disconnect the infusion set and connect the patient to the manometer column

(Reproduced from Sykes (1963), by courtesy of the author and the Editor, Annals of the Royal College of Surgeons)

level (Latimer, 1971; *Figure 24*). Thus the meniscus in the coil at the reference level reflects the venous pressure in the atrium and this can be measured with a low volume displacement device such as an anaeroid pressure gauge or a pressure transducer.

Pressure measurement.—The usual apparatus for measuring venous pressure is a saline manometer (*Figure 25*).

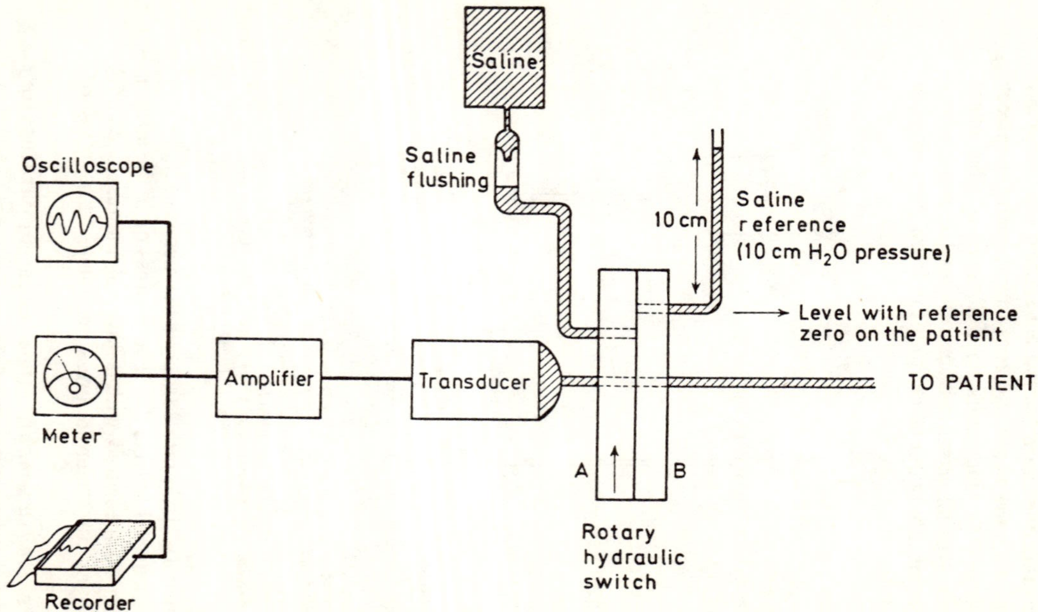

Figure 26. The simplest arrangement for measuring central venous pressure with a pressure transducer and recording system. The reference column of saline is necessary to ensure that alterations in the transducer or amplifier during use do not cause false readings. In its present position the rotary hydraulic switch is connecting the catheter in the patient to the transducer. This is the normal recording position. If A is moved one stop against the arrow, the saline flushes the catheter. If A is moved one stop with the arrow, the saline fills the saline reference. If A is moved one further stop the transducer is connected to the saline reference, which then allows the oscilloscope, meter and recorder to be calibrated. Most systems will also have a position for zero pressure to the transducer

It is simple and it is cheap enough to be disposable, thus removing any risk of cross-infection. Pressure transducers are used (*Figure 26*) but have the disadvantage that they are electrical and—linked as they are to the patient by a conducting liquid column—an electrical fault could cause cardiac arrest with an extremely small current (Monks, 1971). Battery units such as that described by Latimer (1971) should avoid this danger. Pressure transducers have several other disadvantages: they are difficult to sterilize, they are more expensive and more likely to fail than simple saline manometers, and in common with all electrical amplifiers the pressure reading may drift away from the true value because of small changes in the amplifier during operation. However, they are preferred by some because of their faster response to changes in pressure (Jay and Cohn, 1970). If it is necessary to obtain an estimate of the left atrial pressure, an electronic system with a pressure transducer must be used. Direct measurements of left atrial pressure can be made with a simple manometer but measurements of other parameters which are used for indirectly estimating left atrial pressure—such as pulmonary artery end-diastolic pressure—require a more rapidly responding recording system to give accurate readings.

The Evaluation of CVP

Assessment

In the resting normal adult the pressure in the right atrium referred to the mid-right atrial level (Robson, 1968) is 7.7 ± 1.5 cm H_20 (mean $\pm$ SD). The normal left atrial pressure is generally about 5.3 ± 2.7 cm H_2O higher and never lower than the pressure in the right atrium (Braunwald, 1961).

The pressure in the right atrium is low at birth. It is about 0.0 cm H_2O (mid axillary reference) but may be 5 cm H_2O higher if a large placental transfusion has occurred (Burnard and James, 1963; Jegier, Blankenship and Lind, 1963). The effect of the placental transfusion on the right atrial pressure is largely dissipated within 4 hours after birth. The atrial pressure is lower than that in the adult and this may be partly the result of higher intrapleural negative pressures in the newborn. The right atrial pressure swings vary widely with respiration: swings between 5 and 13 cm H_2O were noted in 32 infants 1–31 hours old by Cottom and Young (1965). Again, in infants, left atrial pressure is normally slightly greater than right by about 2 cm H_2O (Rudolph *et al.*, 1961; Burnard and James, 1963).

Factors Affecting the Normal Range

Once a reliable reading has been obtained, it must be compared with the normal range for the situation.

Intrathoracic pressure.—Two factors have an important effect on the normal range. The first is the intrathoracic pressure; any increase in this must increase the pressure immediately outside the ventricles and hence affect the ventricular filling pressure. This is most obvious when the chest is opened and the normal negative intrathoracic pressure is lost (*Figure 27*). A similar effect occurs during intermittent positive pressure ventilation when the inflation pressure increases the mean intrathoracic pressure. A more serious situation occurs in cardiac tamponade when a positive pressure outside the ventricles reduces ventricular filling pressure. Also the liquid in the pericardial sac distends the pericardium which is then less compliant and resists further stretching during ventricular filling. Together these two factors severely reduce ventricular filling. Small increases in intrathoracic pressure can be offset by increases in venous tone (Watson *et al.*, 1962) which tend to maintain the pressure gradients between the peripheral veins and the right atrium, and from the right atrium across the right ventricle. The increase in intrathoracic pressure is transmitted to the pulmonary circulation, left atrium, and left ventricle, so that the pressure gradients tend not to be disturbed on the left side.

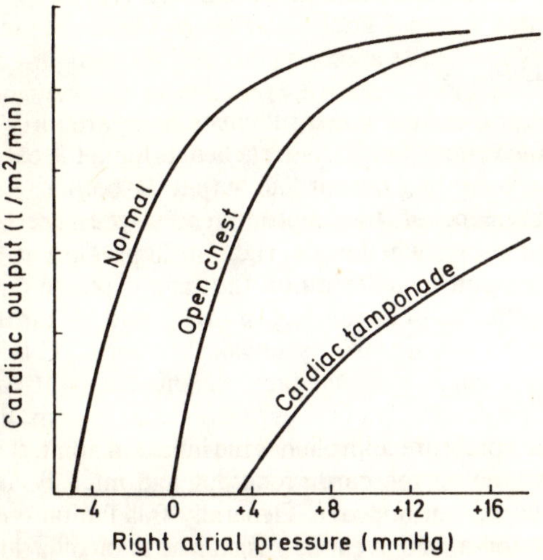

Figure 27. Diagram of cardiac performance under three different conditions of pericardial pressure. Loss of the normal negative intrathoracic pressure shifts the whole curve uniformly to the right, but it is otherwise unchanged. With fluid in the pericardial sac, the curve is shifted still further but is also flattened as ventricular compliance is effectively diminished

(Reproduced from Guyton (1963), by courtesy of the author and the American Physiological Society)

Reference level.—The second factor affecting the normal range is the reference level. The normal central venous pressure range for the chosen reference level must be decided with regard to the patient's position. With a sternal reference point the normal range when a patient is supine is very different to the range when he is prone.

Both of these factors must be estimated and the value for the normal right atrial pressure adjusted accordingly. The probable range of error of these estimates must also be taken into consideration. In most clinical circumstances, this means that even the best conditions give a normal range as wide as 6 cm H_2O. Any failure to assess the prevailing conditions carefully will broaden this range still further.

Interpretation

If the cardiac output is insufficient, there are three possible causes: the venous return has reached its limit, the cardiac performance is limiting the cardiac output, or both.

Measurement of the central venous pressure can help because it shows whether the right atrial pressure is below or above the point of inflexion on the venous return curve. The inflexion point between −4 mmHg and 0 mmHg (approximately) is governed by physical factors and is independent of any cardiovascular factors. This means it can be estimated independently of the cardiovascular system. If the central venous pressure approaches the inflexion point, the venous return is limiting the cardiac output and must be improved before output can improve. Generally this limitation is more the result of a high venous resistance than of a low mean systemic pressure, as normally the baroreceptors ensure maximum sympathetic activity and thus a high mean systemic pressure in a low output state. The high venous resistance is the result of a low venous volume. Restoring blood volume reduces the venous resistance and, with the aid of the sympathetic activity on the veins, restores the mean systemic pressure. This is the basis for the rule of thumb that a central venous pressure below normal means the blood volume is low and volume expansion is indicated. However, spinal anaesthesia or toxins (Knisely *et al.,* 1970) can block venous tone and, without reducing blood volume, reduce the mean systemic pressure to produce a low output state limited by the venous return. In many of these patients, mean systemic pressure and cardiac output can still be restored by increasing the blood volume (Smith and Moore, 1962). Even in uncomplicated haemorrhagic shock it may be necessary to increase the blood volume above normal (MacLean *et al.*, 1965) to maintain the mean systemic pressure and venous return.

If the central venous pressure is well above the normal range, cardiac output is being limited by cardiac performance. The cardiac output can be improved in a number of ways, the simplest of which is to reduce cardiac work to a minimum by keeping the arterial resistance as low as possible. This can be done by alpha-blockade (phenoxybenzamine; Anderson *et al.*, 1967) but the mean systemic pressure will also fall as the venous tone is reduced; thus blood volume may need boosting to restore the mean systemic pressure. A preferred alternative is to give isoprenaline. This reduces arterial resistance and simultaneously increases sympathetic stimulation, thus raising the cardiac performance curve if it is not already maximal. An infusion of isoprenaline has been recommended as a reliable test in haemodynamic problems (MacLean and Duff, 1965). It must be used cautiously, however, as it can produce troublesome arrhythmias (Berk *et al.*, 1972). Digitalis preparations would seem preferable if the peripheral resistance is low and the sympathetic activity high—as indicated by a rapid pulse rate (Cohn *et al.*, 1968). The final criteria are improved cardiac output and tissue perfusion (Carey *et al.*, 1967).

Various drugs have been used in shock—isoprenaline (Shoemaker and Brown, 1971), phenoxybenzamine (Wilson *et al.*, 1964), digoxin (Siegel *et al.*, 1967), and large doses (30 mg/Kg body weight) of steroids (Schumer, 1969; Motsay *et al.*, 1970). Low cardiac output states resulting from cardiac failure or myocardial infarction may be improved by administration of glucagon (Diamond *et al.*, 1971; Amsterdam *et al.*, 1970; Timmis *et al.*, 1973). In septic shock propranolol has been used to reduce vasodilatation (Berk *et al.*, 1972); however, the associated cardiac sympathetic blockade reduces cardiac output and detracts from any advantage gained in the periphery. Here metaraminol does not appear to help but isoprenaline has been recommended (Kardos, 1966). In low output states after myocardial infarction, no benefit is gained from noradrenaline (Cronin, Moore and Marpole, 1965), methoxamine, phenylephrine, or angiotensin (Shubin and Weil, 1967). Furthermore, metaraminol (Smith *et al.*, 1967) and noradrenaline (Friedman *et al.*, 1966) fail to improve the situation significantly in any form of shock (Sambhi *et al.*, 1964). Indeed, vasoconstrictor drugs may confuse the situation by elevating the central venous pressure by 10 cm H_2O or more even when there is a major deficit in blood volume (James and Myers, 1972). The only reports of a beneficial effect of a vasopressor are by Misra and Kezdi (1973) who used a combination of noradrenaline and isoprenaline in low cardiac output states after myocardial infarction and by Wilson, Jablonski and Thal (1964), who combined noradrenaline and phenoxybenzamine in various shock states.

A patient in severe shock or in shock which has failed to respond to treatment, requires careful assessment of his peripheral and cardiac status. His blood pressure, central venous pressure, ECG, urine output and other fluid losses should be monitored closely. Other features of the cardiovascular system may also need to be observed; for example, the left atrial pressure can be observed directly by an atrial catheter or indirectly by a catheter measuring pulmonary wedge pressure. Such detailed examination of the cardiovascular performance is best done in an intensive care or shock unit. From this examination the reason for the shocked state of the patient should become apparent and the treatment of choice should be clear. However the crucial test is that the treatment should be effective. This means that the effect of treatment must be observed critically and closely until the shock has resolved completely. A special unit set up to assess and treat patients in shock can provide a logical approach with gratifying success (Hardaway *et al.*, 1967).

The patients who are most difficult to manage are those who have an obviously low cardiac output but a central venous pressure that is within the estimated normal range. Various authors (Sykes, 1963; Weil, 1969) have advocated a fluid load to test the cardiac performance: an adult is usually given 100–200 ml of fluid intravenously at a rate of 20–60 ml/min. A rise in central venous pressure of more than 3 cm H_2O that persists (*Figure 28*) indicates that the heart cannot handle the increased fluid and that the low output is due to an impaired cardiac performance. An alternative approach has been to try to improve the cardiac performance with isoprenaline (MacLean and Duff, 1965); in this case a fall in central venous pressure indicates a better cardiac performance and therefore

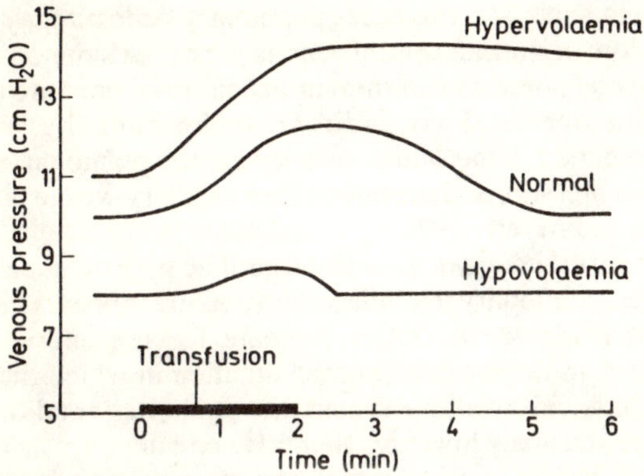

Figure 28. Diagram of the effect of a fluid load to test different situations. In hypovolaemia the fluid causes a brief rise in central venous pressure. Normally there is a modest rise which has vanished by about six minutes. In hypervolaemia the fluid load causes a greater rise in pressure and this rise is more sustained

(Reproduced from Sykes (1963), by courtesy of the author and the Editor, Annals of the Royal College of Surgeons)

a retrospective diagnosis of some cardiac deficiency can be made. The ultimate objective with any test is, however, to improve cardiac output.

The measurement of central venous pressure is less reliable when it is used as an isolated protection against over-infusion (Cooperman and Price, 1970). It may be totally misleading when the 'single pump' approach is inadequate and the left ventricle is so impaired that it requires a high atrial pressure to pump adequately. In this situation pulmonary oedema may occur with only a small change in central venous pressure

(Collins *et al.,* 1971). Old age, a history of cardiac disease, or prolonged cardiovascular insufficiency such as persistent shock, would make it unwise to assume the state of the left ventricle to be adequate. Indeed some workers suggest the compliance of the left ventricle is severely impaired to about one-third of normal when the filling pressure of the left ventricle is chronically elevated by disease (Parker, Khaja and Case, 1970). In such circumstances pulmonary oedema may occur with a low or normal central venous pressure (Simmons *et al.,* 1969b) and some way of measuring left atrial pressure should be considered. Two indirect techniques have been recommended in this situation: they are the pulmonary artery diastolic pressure and the pulmonary capillary wedge pressure (James and Myers, 1972).

Left atrial assessment.—If the cardiac performance is normal the pulmonary end-diastolic pressure appears to be a reliable guide to the filling pressure for the left ventricle. However, in the more important situation in which the filling pressure is chronically elevated, the pulmonary end-diastolic pressure is usually lower by 10 mmHg and does not always increase if the left ventricular filling pressure is increased acutely (Bouchard, Gault and Ross, 1970). Thus a pulmonary arterial end-diastolic pressure measurement seems here to be an unreliable guide to left atrial pressure just when it would be most useful. The pulmonary arterial end-diastolic/left atrial pressure relationship is less close when the pulmonary vascular resistance is high such as in some chronic cardiac states (Jenkins, Bradley and Branthwaite, 1970).

Pulmonary wedge pressure measurements appear to be the most reliable indirect estimates of left atrial pressure (Lappas *et al.,* 1973). This can now be measured with a small, thin disposable catheter. The catheter is light and flexible and so follows the natural flow of the blood from the right heart into the pulmonary artery. The tip lodges in a small peripheral pulmonary artery and the artery can be occluded by the small balloon near the tip (*Figure 29*). This flow-directed catheter can be inserted without fluoroscopy (Ganz *et al.,* 1970). Because the wedge technique occludes the artery, wedge pressure readings should be a good guide to the pressures distal to the catheter; that is, the pulmonary venous and left atrial pressures. These light catheters have been used for monitoring for as long as 3 days (Cerra, Milch and Lajos, 1973).

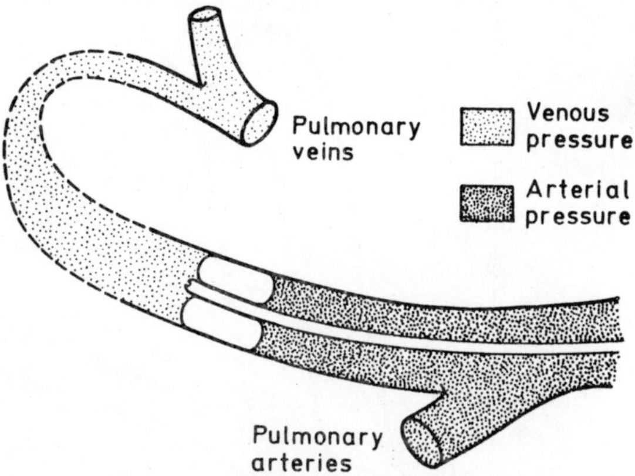

Figure 29. Diagram of a flow-directed catheter in a peripheral pulmonary artery. The small balloon just behind the tip occludes the artery. The lumen of the catheter is open at its tip and thus pressures beyond the inflated balloon can be measured. Under ideal conditions, when there is a low resistance and no anastomoses, this pressure should be almost the same as that in the pulmonary veins and the left atrium. When the balloon is deflated the pulmonary arterial pressure in the periphery is measured

Paediatric use.—If the cardiac state is normal the observation of progressive changes in central venous pressure provides a useful guide to fluid overload, since the right and left atrial pressures increase together. It is for this reason that central venous pressure monitoring has been used during neonatal exchange transfusion (Cottom and Young, 1965) and during fluid replacement in children suffering from severe dehydration (Turcanu, 1972). In very young children who require central venous pressure monitoring it may be necessary to do an elaborate cut-down to the external jugular vein with a skin tunnel to give an exit for the catheter at a site behind the **ear** (Liebert, 1971).

Pulmonary oedema.—The increases in atrial pressure are usually unequal and most figures suggest that the left atrial

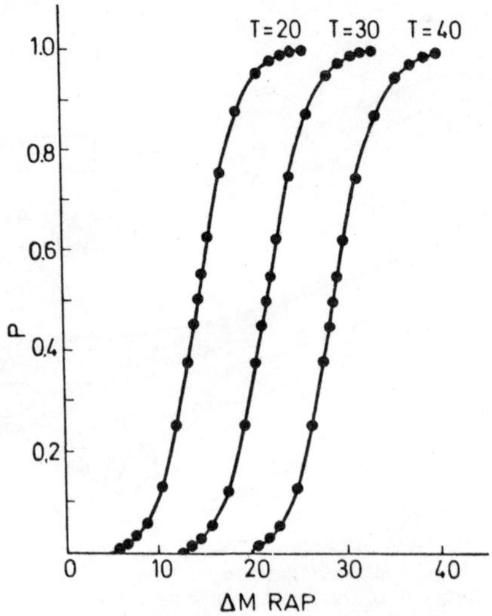

Figure 30. Graph of the probability that a given left atrial pressure (T = 20, 30 or 40 mmHg) will be exceeded by a fluid load producing a certain increase in right atrial pressure (Δ M RAP). Thus for an increase of 21 mmHg in RAP, there is a probability of 0.5 that the left atrial pressure will have exceeded 30 mmHg

(Reproduced from Moss *et al.* (1969), by courtesy of the authors and the Editor, Annals of Surgery)

pressure rises $1\frac{1}{2}$ to 2 times more than the right (figures from Hudspeth and Cordell, 1966; Kerr and Kirklin, 1970; Moss *et al.*, 1969 at P (probability) = 0.5—*Figure 30*). On this basis measurement of the central venous pressure has been used to anticipate pulmonary oedema. If the normal right atrial pressure is 6 cm H_2O and the normal left atrial pressure is 8 cm H_2O, a minimal increase in right atrial pressure can be calculated if we make some broad assumptions. We can reasonably assume that the left atrial rise would not be more than twice that of the right. Moss *et al.,* (1969) showed the probability of this to be very small in baboons, and the investigations of Freitas *et al.* (1965) in man gave a mean ratio of 1:1 for an increase and 1:1.6 for a reduction in circulating blood volume; hence a ratio 1:2 for increments between right and left atrial pressures is probably a cautious estimate for a normal heart. Guyton and Lindsey (1959) suggested that the level of left atrial pressure at which pulmonary oedema may occur is 28 mmHg (38 cm H_2O) or 24 mmHg depending on the reference level. This may be a little high as Forrester, Diamond and McHugh (1971) observed that pulmonary congestion as assessed by radiograph occurred with pulmonary wedge pressures greater than 18 mmHg (24 cm H_2O) in patients with acute myocardial infarction. However, their reference level may have been about 5 mm higher. If a figure of 24 mmHg is accepted, this means a rise in left atrial pressure of some 30 cm H_2O would be required and this would correspond to a rise in right atrial pressure of more than 15 cm H_2O. Certainly a rise of 15 cm H_2O would seem safe as there were no complications when Rubin and Bongiovi (1970) pushed central venous pressure up as much as this to maintain a good urinary output in patients who were suffering from burns. The judicious use of central venous pressure measurement in patients with normal cardiac function can help to prevent over-transfusion and pulmonary oedema (Andersen and Klebe, 1968a).

Clinical Summary

In clinical practice the central venous or right atrial pressure can be used to detect changes in blood volume if a stable baseline is known. It provides a useful estimate of right ventricular function and gives a reliable measure of the balance between systemic venous return and right ventricular performance during transfusion and drug therapy. It does not always rise above the normal level when pulmonary oedema occurs—a point that is particularly relevant if left ventricular performance is impaired by disease, hypoxia, or toxins.

The normal range for the central venous pressure must be carefully estimated with particular regard to the hydrostatic pressure difference between the chosen reference level and the level of the tricuspid valve, and any change in the mean intrathoracic pressure from normal. When there is a low cardiac output the central venous pressure can provide a guide to therapy. An equivocal level of central venous pressure can be tested with a fluid load or isoprenaline. The ultimate criteria of the value of any test are that the test should lead to improved cardiac output and tissue perfusion.

References

Alexander, R. S. (1963). 'The Peripheral Venous System.' In *Handbook of Physiology,* Section 2, Vol. 2, Chap. 31. Washington; American Physiological Society.

Amsterdam, E. A., Zelis, R., Spann, J. F., Hurley, E. J. and Mason, D. T. (1970). 'Cardiocirculatory Effects of Glucagon in Patients with Congestive Heart Failure and Cardiogenic Shock.' *Am. J. Cardiol.,* **25,** 82. (Abstr.)

Andersen, D. and Klebe, J. G. (1968a). 'Report of Experiences in 142 Patients with Gastro-intestinal Bleeding Requiring Transfusion.' *Scand, J. Gastroenterol.,* **3,** 113–122.

Andersen, D. and Klebe, J. G. (1968b). 'Measurement of C.V.P. Complications and Possible Failures of the Method.' *Scand. J. Gastroenterol.*, **3,** 267–272.

Anderson, R. W., James, P. M., Bredenberg, C. E. and Hardaway, R. M. (1967). 'Phenoxybenzamine in Septic Shock.' *Ann. Surg.*, **165,** 341–350.

Aubaniac, R. (1952). 'L'injection intraveineuse sous-claviculaire: Advantages et Technique.' *Presse méd.*, **60,** 1456.

Banet, M. and Guyton, A. C. (1971). 'Effect of Body Metabolism on Cardiac Output: Role of the Central Nervous System.' *Am. J. Physiol.*, **220,** 662–666.

Bansmer, G., Keith, D. and Tesluk, H. (1958). 'Complications Following use of Indwelling Catheters in the Inferior Vena Cava.' *J. Amer. med. Ass.*, **167,** 1606–1611.

Barrat-Boyes, B. G. and Wood, E. H. (1957). 'The Oxygen Saturation of Blood in the Venae Cavae, Right Heart Chambers and Pulmonary Vessels of Healthy Subjects.' *J. Lab. clin. Med.*, **50,** 93–106.

Benchimol, A. (1969). 'Significance of the Contribution of Atrial Systole to Cardiac Function in Man.' *Am. J. Cardiol.*, **23,** 568–571.

Berglund, E. (1954). 'Ventricular Function VI Balance of Left and Right Ventricular Output: Relation between Left and Right Atrial Pressures.' *Am. J. Physiol.*, **178,** 381–386.

Berk, J. L. Hagen, J. F., Maly, G. and Koo, R. (1972). 'The Treatment of Shock with Beta Adrenergic Blockade.' *Archs Surg., Chicago*, **104,** 46–51.

Bernard, R. W. and Stahl, W. M. (1971). 'Subclavian Vein Catheterization: A Prospective Study. I. Non-infectious Complications.' *Ann. Surg.*, **173,** 184–190.

Bishop, V. S. and Stone, H. L. (1967). 'Quantitative Description of Ventricular Output Curves in Conscious Dogs.' *Circulat. Res.*, **20,** 581–586.

Bouchard, R. J., Gault, J. H. and Ross, J. (1970). 'Evaluation of Pulmonary Arterial End-diastolic Pressure as an Estimate of Left Ventricular End-diastolic pressure in Patients with Acute and Chronic Alterations in Left Ventricular Performance.' *Am. J. Cardiol.*, **25,** 86. (Abstr.)

Bradley, E. C. (1965). 'Results with Phentolamine (Regitine) in the Treatment of Selected Patients with Shock.' *Calif. Med.*, **103,** 314–315.

Bradley, R. D., Jenkins, B. S. and Branthwaite, M. A. (1970). 'The Influence of Atrial Pressure on Cardiac Performance following Myocardial Infarction Complicated by Shock.' *Circulation*, **42,** 827–837.

Brandt, R. L., Foley, W. J., Fink, G. H. and Regan, W. J. (1970).

'Mechanism of Perforation of the Heart with Production of Hydropericardium by a Venous Catheter and its Prevention.' *Am. J. Surg.*, **119**, 311–316.

Braunwald, E., Brockenbrough, E. C., Frahm, C. J. and Ross, J. (1961). 'Left Atrial and Left Ventricular Pressures in Subjects without Cardiovascular Disease. Observations in Eighteen Patients Studied by Trans-septal Left Heart Catheterization.' *Circulation,* **24,** 267–269.

– and Ross, J. (1964). 'Applicability of Starling's Law of the Heart to Man.' *Circulation Res.,* **15,** Suppl. 2, 169–178.

Briscoe, C. E. (1973). 'A Comparison of Jugular and Central Venous Pressure Measurements During Anaesthesia.' *Br. J. Anaesth.,* **45,** 173–178.

Brobmann, G. F., Klano, H. B., Moore, G., Meyer, P., Breecher, G. A. and Jacobson, E. D. (1971). 'Effect of Acute Haemorrhage on Arterial and Venous Resistance.' *Am. J. Physiol.,* **220,** 12–15.

Burnard, E. D. and James, L. S. (1963). 'Atrial Pressures and Cardiac Size in the Newborn Infant.' *J. Pediat.,* **62,** 815–826.

Campeau, L., Pospisil, L., Grondin, P., Dyrda, I. and Lepage, G. (1970). 'Cardiac Catheter Findings at Rest and after Exercise in Patients following Cardiac Transplantation.' *Am. J. Cardiol.,* **25,** 523–528.

Carey, J. S., Mohr, P. A., Brown, R. S. and Shoemaker, W. C. (1969). 'Cardiovascular Function in Haemorrhage Trauma and Sepsis: Determinants of Cardiac Output and Work.' *Ann. Surg.,* **170,** 910–921.

— Brown, R. S., Mohr, P. A., Monson, D. O., Yao, S. T. and Shoemaker, W. C. (1967). 'Cardiovascular Function in Shock. Responses to Volume Loading and Isoproterenol Infusion.' *Circulation,* **35,** 327–338.

Cerra, F., Milch, R. and Lajos, T. Z. (1973). 'Pulmonary Artery Catheterization in Critically Ill Surgical Patients.' *Ann. Surg.,* **177,** 37–39.

Clarke-Kennedy, A. E. (1929). *Stephen Hales D.D. F.R.S.* London; Cambridge University Press.

Cohn, J. D., Greenspan, M., Goldstein, C. R., Gudwin, A. L., Siegel, J. H. and Del Guercio, L. R. M. (1968). 'Arteriovenous Shunting in High Cardiac Output Shock Syndromes.' *Surgery Gynec. Obstet.,* **127,** 282–288.

Cohnheim, J. and Lichtheim, L. (1877). 'Ueber Hydrämie und Hydrämisches Oedem.' *Virchows Arch. path. Anat. Physiol.,* **69,** 106–143.

Colditz, R. B. (1970). 'Central Venous Pressure in Supine Position during Normal Pregnancy. Comparative Determinations during First, Second and Third Trimesters.' *Obstet. Gynec., N.Y.,* **36,** 769–772.

Collins, J. V., Clark, T. J. H., Evans, T. R. and Riaz, M. A. (1971). 'Central Venous Pressure in Acute Myocardial Infarction.' *Lancet,* **1,** 373–375.

Cooperman, L. H. and Price, H. L. (1970). 'Pulmonary Edema in the Operative and Postoperative Period.' *Ann. Surg.,* **172,** 883–891.

Cottom, D. and Young, M. (1965). 'Venous Pressure Measurement in Exchange Transfusion.' *Archs. Dis. Childh.,* **40,** 323.

Cournand, A. R., Riley, R. L., Bradley, S. E., Bried, E. S., Noble, R. P., Lauson, H. D., Gregersen, M. I. and Richards, D. W. (1943). 'Studies of the Circulation in Clinical Shock.' *Surgery, St. Louis,* **13,** 964.

Cronin, R. F. P., Moore, S. and Marpole, D. G. (1965). 'Shock following Myocardial Infarction: a Clinical Survey of 140 Cases.' *Canad. med. Ass. J.,* **93,** 57.

Crowell, J. W. (1970). 'Oxygen Transport in the Hypotensive State.' *Fedn. Proc.,* **29,** 1848–1853.

Davidson, J. T., Ben Hur, N. and Nathen, H. (1963). 'Subclavian Venipuncture (Infraclavicular).' *Lancet,* **2,** 1139–1140.

DeBrunner, F. and Bühler, F. (1969). '"Normal C.V.P.", the Significance of the Reference Point and the Normal Range,' *Br. med. J.,* **3,** 148–150.

Diamond, G., Forrester, J., Danzig, R., Parmley, W. W. and Swan, H. J. C. (1971). 'Haemodynamic Effects of Glucagon during Acute Myocardial Infarction with Left Ventricular Failure in Man.' *Br. Heart J.,* **33,** 290–295.

Diem, K. and Lentner, C. (Eds.) (1970). *Geigy Scientific Tables,* 7th ed., p. 557. Basle; Geigy.

Doty, D. B. (1969). 'The Practical Value of the Central Venous Catheter for Monitoring the Patient in Shock.' *J. Trauma,* **9,** 148–149.

Dykes, M. H. M. and Fuller, J. E. (1969). 'Post-transfusion Pulmonary Edema in Surgical Patients: Etiology and Therapeutic Use of Trimetaphan Camphorsulfonate (Arfonad).' *Anesthesiology,* **30,** 101–106.

English, I. C. W., Frew, R. M., Piggott, J. F. and Zaki, M. (1969). 'Percutaneous Catheterization of the Internal Jugular Vein.' *Anaesthesia,* **24,** 521–531.

Eustace, B. R. (1970). 'A Comparison between Peripheral and Central Venous Pressure Monitoring under Clinical Conditions.' *Injury,* **2,** 14–18.

Forrester, J. S., Diamond, G. and McHugh, T. J. (1971). 'Filling Pressure in the Right and Left Sides of the Heart in Acute Myocardial Infarction. A Re-appraisal of Central Venous Pressure Monitoring.' *New Engl. J. Med.,* **285,** 190–193.

Freitas, F. M. De., Faraco, E. Z., Azevedo, D. F. de, Zaduchliver, J. and Lewin, I. (1965). 'Behavior of Normal Pulmonary Circulation during Changes of Total Blood Volume in Man.' *J. clin. Invest.*, **44**, 366–378.

Friedman, E., Grable, E. and Fine, J. (1966). 'Central Venous Pressure and Direct Serial Measurements as Guides in Blood Volume Replacement.' *Lancet*, **2**, 609–614.

Fry, R. L., Braunwald, E. and Cohen, E. R. (1960). 'Studies on Starling's Law of the Heart. I. The Circulatory Response to Acute Hypervolemia and its Modification by Ganglion Blockade.' *J. clin. Invest.*, **39**, 1043–1050.

Gaar, K. A., Taylor A. E., Owens, L. J. and Guyton, A. C. (1967). 'Effects of Capillary Pressure and Plasma Proteins on the Development of Pulmonary Edema.' *Am. J. Physiol.*, **213**, 79–82.

Ganz, W. W., Forrester, J. S., Chonette, D., Donoso, R. and Swan, H. J. C. (1970). 'A New Flow-directed Catheter Technique for Measurement of Pulmonary Artery and Capillary Wedge Pressure without Fluoroscopy.' *Am. J. Cardiol.*, **25**, 96. (Abstr.)

Gilday, D. L. and Downs, A. R. (1969). 'Value of Chest Radiography in Localization of Central Venous Pressure Catheters.' *Can. med. Ass. J.*, **101**, 363–364.

Glick, G., Sonnenblick, E. H. and Braunwald, E. (1965). 'Myocardiac Force-velocity Relations Studied in Intact Unanesthetized Man.' *J. clin. Invest.*, **44**, 978–988.

Goldman, R. H., Klughaupt, M., Metcalf, T., Spivak, A. P. and Harrison, D. C. (1968). 'Measurement of Central Venous Oxygen Saturation in Patients with Myocardial Infarction.' *Circulation*, **38**, 941–946.

Gould, L., Zahir, M., Shariff, M. and Guiliani, M. (1970). 'Phentolamine: use in Pulmonary Edema. Preliminary Report. *Jap. Heart J.*, **11**, 141–148.

Gudwin, A. L., Goldstein, C. R., Cohn, J. D. and Del Guercio, L. R. M. (1967). 'Indicator Dilution Curve Analysis for the Prediction of Operative Mortality in Elderly Patients.' *Surg, Forum*, **18**, 167–170.

Gutierrez, V. S., Berman, I. R., Soloway, H. B. and Hamit, H. F. (1970). 'Relationship of Hypoproteinemia and Prolonged Mechanical Ventilation to the Development of Pulmonary Insufficiency in Shock.' *Ann. Surg.*, **171**, 385–393.

Guyton, A. C. (1963). 'Venous return.' In *Handbook of Physiology*, Section 2, Vol. 2, Chap. 32. Washington; American Physiological Society.

— and Adkins, L. H. (1954). 'Quantitative Aspects of the Collapse Factor in Relation to Venous Return.' *Am. J. Physiol.*, **177**, 523–527.

— and Greganti, F. P. (1956). 'A Physiologic Reference Point for Measuring Circulatory Pressure in the Dog, particularly Venous Pressure.' *Am. J. Physiol.*, **185**, 137–141.

Guyton, A. C. and Lindsey, A. W. (1959). 'Effects of Elevated Left Atrial Pressure and Decreased Plasma Protein Concentration on the Development of Pulmonary Edema.' *Circulat. Res.*, **7,** 649–657.

— and Sagawa, K. (1961), 'Compensation of Cardiac Output and other Circulatory Functions in Areflexic Dogs with Large A-V Fistulae.' *Am. J. Physiol.*, **200,** 1157–1163.

— Lindsey, A. W., Abernathy, B. and Langston, J. B. (1958a). 'Mechanism of the Increased Venous Return and Cardiac Output caused by Epinephrine.' *Am. J. Physiol.*, **192,** 126–130.

— — — and Richardson, T. (1957). 'Venous Return at Various Right Atrial Pressures and the Normal Venous Return Curve.' *Am. J. Physiol.*, **189,** 609–615.

— — Kaufman, N. B. and Abernathy, J. B. (1958b). 'Effect of Blood Transfusion and Hemorrhage on Cardiac Output and on the Venous Return Curve.' *Am. J. Physiol.*, **194,** 263–267.

— — Langston, J. B., Kaufman, B. N. and Fairchild, H. M. (1959). 'Relative Importance of Venous and Arterial Resistances in Controlling Venous Return and Cardiac Output.' *Am. J. Physiol.*, **196,** 1008–1014.

Hainsworth, R. and Karim, F. (1974). 'Changes in Abdominal Vascular Capacity in Response to Stimulation of Efferent Sympathetic Nerves.' *J. Physiol., Lond.*. Proceedings (January).

Hardaway, R. M., James, P. N., Anderson, R. W., Bredenburg, C. E. and West, R. L. (1967). 'Intensive Study and Treatment of Shock in Man.' *J. Amer. med. Ass.*, **199,** 779–790.

Holt, J. P. (1940). 'The Measurement of Venous Pressure in Man Eliminating the Hydrostatic Factor.' *Am. J. Physiol.*, **130,** 635–641.

Howell, W. H. and Donaldson, F. (1884). 'Experiments upon the Heart of the Dog with Reference to the Maximum Volume sent out by the Left Ventricle Beat and the Influence of Variations in Venous Pressure, Arterial Pressure and Pulse Rate upon Work done by the Heart.' *Phil. Trans. R. Soc.*, B, **175,** 139–160.

Hudspeth, A. S. and Cordell, A. R. (1966), 'Cardiovascular Responses to induced Hypervolemia.' *Ann. Surg.*, **164,** 183–189.

Hughes, R. E. and Magovern, G. J. (1959). 'The Relationship between Right Atrial Pressure and Blood Volume.' *Archs Surg.*, **79,** 238–243.

James, P. M. and Myers, R. T. (1972). 'Central Venous Pressure Monitoring: Misinterpretation, Abuses, Indications and a New Technic.' *Ann. Surg.*, **175,** 693–701.

Jay, N. and Cohn, J. G. (1970). 'Monitoring Techniques in Shock.' *Am. J. Cardiol.*, **26,** 565–569.

Jegier, W., Blankenship, W. and Lind, J. (1963). 'Venous Pressure in the First Hour of Life and its Relationship to Placental

Transfusion.' *Acta paediat., Stockh.,* **52,** 485–496.

Jenkins, B. S., Bradley, R. D. and Branthwaite, M. A. (1970). 'Evaluation of Pulmonary Arterial End-diastolic Pressure as an Indirect Estimate of Left Atrial Mean Pressure.' *Circulation,* **42,** 75.

Jones, R. R. (1963). 'Venous Pressure in General Anesthesia.' *Anesth, Analg. curr. Res.,* **42,** 470.

Kardos, G. G. (1966). 'Isoproterenol in the Treatment of Shock due to Bacteremia with Gram Negative Pathogens.' *New Engl. J. Med.,* **274,** 868.

Kellner, G. A. and Smart, J. F. (1972). 'Percutaneous Placement of Catheters to Monitor "Central Venous Pressure".' *Anesthesiology,* **36,** 515–516.

Kerr, A. R. and Kirklin, J. W. (1970). 'Effect of Rapid Increases in Blood Volume on Atrial Pressure and Pulmonary Blood Volume.' *Ann. Surg.,* **172,** 278–283.

Kerr, M. G., Scott, D. B. and Samuel, E. (1964). 'Studies of the Inferior Vena Cava in Late Pregnancy.' *Br. med. J.,* **1,** 532–533.

Knisely, M. H., Cowley, R. A., Hawthorne, I. and Garris, D. (1970). 'Separation of Shock Types.' *Angiology,* **21,** 728–744.

Kuramoto, K. and Rodbard, S. (1962). 'Effects of Blood Flow and Left Atrial Pressure on Pulmonary Venous Resistance.' *Circulation Res.,* **11,** 240–246.

Lappas, D., Lell, W. A., Gabel, J. C., Civetta, J. M. and Lowenstein, E. (1973). 'Indirect Measurement of Left Atrial Pressure in Surgical Patients—Pulmonary-capillary Wedge and Pulmonary-artery Diastolic Pressures compared with Left-atrial Pressure.' *Anesthesiology,* **38,** 394–397.

Latimer, R. D. (1971). 'Central Venous Catheterisation.' *Br. J. Hosp. Med.,* **5,** 369–376.

Leachman, R. D., Cokkinos, D. V. P., Zamalloa, O. and Alvarez, A. (1969). 'Electrocardiographic Behavior of Recipient and Donor Atria after Human Heart Transplant.' *Am. J. Cardiol.,* **24,** 49–53.

— Cabrera, R., Leatherman, L. L. and Rochelle, D. G. (1971). 'Response of the Transplanted Denervated Human Heart to Cardiovascular Drugs.' *Am. J. Cardiol.,* **27,** 272–276.

— Leatherman, L. L., Rochelle, D. G., Cooley, D. A., Hallman, G. L., Bloodwell, R. D. and Nora, J. J. (1969). 'Psysiologic Behavior of the Transplanted Heart in Six Human Recipients.' *Am. J. Cardiol.,* **23,** 123. (Abstr.)

Lee, J., Wright, F., Barber, R. and Stanley, L. (1972). 'Central Venous Oxygen-Saturation in Shock: a Study in Man.' *Anesthesiology,* **36,** 472–478.

Lewin, I., Lerner, A. G., Green, S. H., Del Guercio, L. R. M. and Siegel, J. H. (1971). 'Physical Class and Physiologic Status in the Prediction of Operative Mortality in the Aged Sick.' *Ann. Surg.,*

174, 217–231.

Liebert, P. S. (1971). 'Central Venous Catheters in Children—their Placement and Care.' *Clin. Pediat.,* **10,** 218–222.

MacLean, L. D. and Duff. J. H. (1965). 'The Use of C.V.P. as a Guide to Volume Replacement in Shock.' *Dis. Chest,* **48,** 199–205.

— — Scott, H. M. and Peretz, D. I. (1965). 'Treatment of Shock in Man based on Hemodynamic Diagnosis.' *Surgery Gynec. Obstet.,* **120,** 1–16.

Majid, P. A., Sharma, B. and Taylor, S. H. (1971). 'Phentolamine for Vasodilator Treatment of Severe Heart Failure.' *Lancet,* **2,** 719–724.

Mantle, J. A., Russell, R. O., Dowling, J. T. and Rackley, C. E. (1973). 'The Relationship of Left Ventricular Filling Pressure to Left Ventricular Function in Acute Myocardial Infarction.' *Clin. Res.,* **21,** 38. (Abstr.)

Misra, S. N. and Kezdi, P. (1973). 'Hemodynamic Effects of Adrenergic Stimulating and Blocking Agents in Cardiogenic Shock and Low Output State after Myocardial Infarction.' *Am. J. Cardiol.,* **31,** 724–735.

Mitchell, J. H. and Shapiro, W. (1969). 'Atrial Function and Hemodynamic Consequences of Atrial Fibrillation in Man.' *Am. J. Cardiol.,* **23,** 556–567.

Monks, P. S. (1971). 'Safe use of Electromedical Equipment.' *Anaesthesia,* **26,** 264–280.

Moran, J. M., Atwood, R. P. and Rowe, M. I. (1965). 'A Clinical and Bacteriologic Study of Infection Associated with Venous Cut Downs.' *New Engl. J. Med.,* **272,** 554.

Moss, G. S., Homer, L. D., Herman, C. M. and Proctor, H. J. (1969). 'Right Atrial and Pulmonary Artery Pressure as Indicators of Left Atrial Pressure during Fluid Therapy following Hemorrhagic Shock in the Baboon.' *Ann. Surg.,* **170,** 801–812.

Motsay, G. J. Alho, A., Jaeger, T., Dietzman, R. H. and Lillehei, R. C. (1970). 'Effects of Corticosteroids on the Circulation in Shock: Experimental and Clinical Results.' *Fedn Proc.,* **29,** 1861–1873.

Nunn, J. F. and Freeman, J. (1964). 'Problems of Oxygenation and Oxygen Transport during Haemorrhage.' *Anaesthesia,* **19,** 206–216.

Parikh, R. K. (1972). 'Horner's Syndrome: A Complication of Percutaneous Catheterisation of Internal Jugular Vein.' (case report). *Anaesthesia,* **27,** 327–329.

Parker, J. O., Khaja, F. and Case, R. B. (1970). 'Assessment of Left Ventricular Function in Man through Graded Alterations in Stroke Volume. *Am. J. Cardiol.,* **25,** 120. (Abstr.)

Pedersen, A. and Husby, J. (1951). 'Venous Pressure Measurement 1. Choice of Zero Level.' *Acta med. scand.,* **141,** 185–194.

Ramo, B. W., Myers, N., Wallace, A. G., Starmer, F., Clark, D. O. and Whalen, R. E. (1970). 'Hemodynamic Findings in 123 Patients with Acute Myocardial Infarction on Admission.' *Circulation*, **42**, 567–577.

Robinson, B. F., Epstein, S. E., Kohler, R. L. and Braunwald, E. (1966). 'Circulatory Effects of Acute Expansion of Blood Volume. Studies during Maximal Exercise and at Rest.' *Circulat. Res.*, **19**, 26–32.

Robson, M. C. (1968). 'Reproducible Central Venous Pressure.' *Johns Hopkins med. J.*, **122**, 232–235.

Ross, J. and Braunwald, E. (1964). 'The Study of Left Ventricular Function in Man by Increasing Resistance to Ventricular Ejection with Angiotensin.' *Circulation*, **29**, 739–749.

Rubin, L. R. and Bongiovi, J. (1970). 'Central Venous Pressure, an Unreliable Guide to Fluid Therapy in Burns.' *Archs Surg., Chicago*, **100**, 269–274.

Rudolph, A. M., Drorbaugh, J. E., Auld, P. A. M., Rudolph, A. J., Nadas, A. S., Smith, C. A. and Hubbell, J. P. (1961). 'Studies on the Circulation in the Neonatal Period.' *Pediatrics, Springfield*, **27**, 551–566.

Rushman, G. B., Ferguson, A. and Boulton, T. B. (1970). 'Catheterization of the Superior Vena Cava.' *St. Bart's Hosp. J.*, **74**, 363–368.

Rushmer, R. F. (1959). 'Constancy of Stroke Volume in Ventricular Response to Exertion.' *Am. J. Physiol.*, **196**, 743–750

Russell, R. O., Rackley, C. E., Pombo, J., Hunt, D., Potanin, C. and Dodge, H. T. (1970). 'Effect of Increasing Left Ventricular Filling Pressure in Patients with Acute Myocardial Infarction.' *J. clin. Invest.*, **49**, 1539–1550.

Ryan, G. M. and Howland, W. S. (1966). 'An Evaluation of Central Venous Pressure Monitoring.' *Anesth, Analg. curr. Res.*, **45**, 754–759.

Sambhi, M. P., Weil, M. H., Udhoji, V. N. and Rosoff, L. (1964). 'Effect of Pressor Amines on Cardiac Output on Patients with Acute Hypotension.' *Circulation*, **30**, 485–492.

Sarnoff, S. J. (1955), 'Myocardial Contractility as Described by Ventricular Function Curves: Observations on Starling's Law of the Heart.' *Physiol. Rev.*, **7**, 107–122.

Scheinman, M. M., Brown, M. A. and Rapaport, E. (1969). 'Critical Assessment of use of Central Venous Oxygen Saturation as a Mirror of Mixed Venous Oxygen in Severely Ill Cardiac Patients.' *Circulation*, **40**, 165–172.

Schumer, W. (1969). 'Dexamethasone in Oligemic Shock. Physicochemical Effects in Monkeys.' *Archs Surg., Chicago*, **98**, 259–261.

Seldinger, S. I. (1953). 'Catheter Replacement of the Needle in Percutaneous Arteriography. *Acta radiol.,* **39,** 368–376.

Sharpey-Schafer, E. P. (1963). 'Venous Tone: Effects of Reflex Changes, Humoral Agents and Exercise.' *Br. med. Bull.,* **19,** 145–148.

Shoemaker, W. C. and Brown, R. S. (1971). 'The Dilemma of Vasopressors and Vasodilators in the Therapy of Shock.' *Surgery Gynec. Obstet.,* **132,** 51–57.

Shubin, H. and Weil, M. H. (1967). 'The Treatment of Shock Complicating Acute Myocardial Infarction.' *Prog. cardiovasc. Dis.,* **10,** 30–54.

Siegel, H. W. and Downing, S. E. (1970). 'Reduction of Left Ventricular Contractility during Hemorrhagic Shock.' *Am. J. Physiol.,* **218,** 772–779.

Siegel, J. H., Greenspan, M. and Del Guercio, L. R. M. (1967). 'Abnormal Vascular Tone, Defence Oxygen Transport and Myocardial Failure in Human Septic Shock.' *Ann. Surg.,* **165,** 504–517.

— and Williams, J. B. (1969). 'A Computer based Index for the Prediction of Operative Survival in Patients with Cirrhosis and Portal Hypertension.' *Ann. Surg.,* **169,** 191–201.

Simmons, R. L., Heisterkamp, C. A., Moseley, R. V. and Doty, D. B. (1969a). 'Post-resuscitation Blood Volumes in Combat Casualties.' *Surgery Gynec. Obstet.,* **128,** 1193–1201.

— — Collins, J. A., Bredenburg, C. E. and Martin, A. M. (1969b). 'Acute Pulmonary Edema in Battle Casualties.' *J. Trauma,* **9,** 760–775.

Smith, B. E., Modell, J. H., Gaub, M. L. and Moya, E. (1965). 'Complications of Subclavian Vein Catheterization.' *Archs Surg.,* **90,** 228–229.

Smith, H. J., Oriol, A., Morch, J. and McGregor, M. (1967). 'Hemodynamic Studies in Cardiogenic Shock. Treatment with Isoproterenol and Metaraminol.' *Circulation,* **35,** 1084–1091.

Smith, L. L. and Moore, F. D. (1962). 'Refractory Hypotension in Man—is this Irreversible Shock?' *New Engl. J. Med.,* **267,** 733–742.

Spodick, D. H. (1967). 'Acute Cardiac Tamponade. Pathologic Physiology, Diagnosis and Management.' *Prog. Cardiovasc. Dis.,* **10,** 64–96.

Starling, E. H. (1918). 'The Linacre Lecture on the Law of the Heart.' Given at Cambridge, 1915. London; Longman.

Stoelting, R. K. (1973). 'Evaluation of External Jugular Venous Pressure as a Reflection of Right Atrial Pressure.' *Anesthesiology,* **38,** 291–294.

Stone, A. M. and Stahl, W. M. (1970). 'Renal Effects of Hemorrhage in Normal Man.' *Ann, Surg.,* **172,** 825–836.

Swaroop, S. (1972). 'Knotting of Two Central Venous Monitoring Catheters.' *Am. J. Med.,* **53,** 386–388.

Sykes, M. K. (1963). 'Venous Pressure as a Clinical Indication of Adequacy of Transfusion.' *Ann. R. Coll. Surg.*, **33,** 185–197.

Taylor, D. E. M. (1972). 'Computation of Cardiac Function Curves during Surgery.' *Proc. R. Soc. Med.*, **65,** 891. (Abstr.)

Thomas, C. S., Carter, J. W. and Lowder, S. C, (1969). 'Pericardial Tamponade from Central Venous Catheters.' *Archs Surg.*, **98,** 217–218.

Thomasson, B. (1959). 'A Study in Right Heart Performance in Man with Special Reference to the Effects of Experimentally Induced Acute Hypervolemia.' *Scand, J. clin. Lab. Invest.*, **11,** Suppl. 40. 1–76.

Timmis, G. C., Lin, R., Ramos, R. G. and Gordon, S. (1973). 'Prolonged Glucagon Infusion in Cardiac Failure.' *J. Amer. med. Ass.*, **223,** 293–296.

Turcanu, L. (1972). 'Usefulness of Measurement of Central Venous Pressure in Acute Dehydration Syndrome in Infants.' *Pediatria Buc.* **21,** 269–274.

Turner, D. D. and Sommers, S. C. (1954). 'Accidental Passage of Polyethylene Catheter from Cubital Vein to Right Atrium.' *New Engl. J. Med.*, **251,** 744.

Visscher, M. B., Haddy, F. J. and Stephens, G. (1956). 'The Physiology of Lung Edema.' *Pharmac. Rev.*, **8,** 389–434.

Wartman, W. B. and Kellerstein, H. K. (1948). 'Incidence of Heart Disease in 2,000 Consecutive Autopsies.' *Ann. intern, Med.*, **28,** 41–65.

Watson, W. E., Smith, A. C. and Spalding, J. M. K. (1962). 'Transmural Central Venous Pressure during Intermittent Positive Pressure Respirations.' *Br. J. Anaesth.*, **34,** 278–286.

Webre, D. R. and Arens,J. F. (1973). 'Use of Cephalic and Basilic Veins for Introduction of Central Venous Catheters.' *Anesthesiology,* **38,** 389–392.

Weil, M. H. (1969). 'Progress in the Bedside Management of Shock.' *J. Trauma,* **9,** 154–156.

Wilson, R. F., Jablonski, D. V. and Thal, A. P. (1964). 'The Usage of Dibenzyline in Clinical Shock.' *Surgery, St Louis,* **56,** 172–183.

Winsor, T. and Burch, G. E. (1945). 'Phlebostatic Axis and Phlebostatic Level. Reference Levels for Venous Pressure in Man.' *Proc. Soc. exp. Biol. Med.*, **58,** 165–169.

Wood, P. (1968). *Diseases of the Heart and Circulation,* 3rd ed., p. 620. London; Eyre and Spottiswoode.

Woods, D. G., Lumley, J., Russell, W. J. and Jack, R. D. (1974). 'The Position of Central Venous Catheters Inserted through Arm Veins: A Preliminary Report.' *Anaesth. Intens. Care,* **2.** (In Press).

Yoffa, D. (1965). 'Supraclavicular Subclavian Venipuncture and Catheterization.' *Lancet,* **2,** 614–617.

Index